About the Author

Kay was born and bred in L[...] town. Her life was just a nor[...] independent and determined [...] made her rescue mice from [...] also set off mouse traps wh[...] poor mouse family from more [...]

C000193480

[...]n a [...]een [...]hat [...]he [...]the

As a child, she went to school at the local girls grammar school and left at 16 to start a pre-nursing course. She met her husband Philip at 17 and was married at 18. She soon discovered that training was impractical for her circumstances and, instead, took a position in a bank and saved for England!

At 21, Kay and her husband bought a fish and chip shop and while running that, Philip ran his engineering business: in her spare time, Kay kept Philip's accounts; in his spare time, Philip helped fry fish and chips. It was hectic time, but both were young and didn't understand the term "burning the candle from both ends".

At 22, Kay's first child was born and the next year the fish and chip shop was sold. Three more children followed in quick succession until by the age of 27, the author was the proud mother of four children under the age of five! She still kept the accounts although she did take two years off after the birth of her fourth child.

As the children grew, life was busy and Kay was often tired but put it down to being a mum. At the age of 35, however, Kay began feeling very ill and at 37 suffered a heart attack. It wasn't until she was 38 that Kay knew it was all because of Hughes Syndrome.

Since that time, Kay has been writing books and helping others via the internet, and this has been her main drive in life; as her husband says "it's her thing". She still helps her husband with his business, and now has four young adults to guide through life.

Despite life's ups and downs Kay feels blessed by all that she has. Illness is life changing but once you learn to live with it life is still great!

More Sticky Blood

by

Kay Thackray

Published 2005 by arima publishing

www.arimapublishing.com

ISBN 1-84549-061-4

© Kay Thackray 2005

Printed and bound in the United Kingdom

Typeset in Verdana 10/14

arima publishing
ASK House, Northgate Avenue
Bury St Edmunds, Suffolk IP32 6BB
t: (+44) 01284 700321

www.arimapublishing.com

*This book is dedicated to
Philip Thackray,
whose example has taught me to
never give up whatever the odds may be.*

*I would like to thank all of those involved in the research and
treatment of this illness. Without their work both myself and
many others would be unable to live productive and happy
lives.
They have helped many of us just to be alive.*

Thank you doesn't really cover that, does it?

Preface
by Dr Graham R V Hughes MD FRCP

Although it is over twenty years since Hughes syndrome was described, it is clear that many, many patients go undiagnosed.

As the 'sticky blood' phenomenon of Hughes syndrome can affect every organ, it is not uncommon for a patient to be seen by a variety of doctors – a cardiologist for chest pain, for example, a neurologist for suspected multiple sclerosis, a general practitioner for fatigue and aches and pains – all possibly missing clinical clues such as the long history of migraine, the miscarriages 15 years previously, the memory loss and difficulty in finding words, the family history of stroke and thrombosis...

In her first book (Sticky Blood Explained), Kay Thackray highlighted these problems in a vividly clear and graphic account of Hughes syndrome seen from a patient's perspective.

In this, her second book on the syndrome, Kay Thackray gives valuable insights and advice on living with the syndrome.

It is a fact that many patients find great comfort from comparing notes with others with similar problems. For this reason alone, I believe that More Sticky Blood will do more than a library full of medical texts to help Hughes syndrome patients overcome their disease.

Dr Graham R V Hughes MD FRCP
Consultant Rheumatologist
St. Thomas' Hospital, London

Contents

Preface   vii

Introduction   11

Chapter 1 -   Those endless tests and how   13
              to survive them.

Chapter 2 -   The very first Hughes Syndrome   25
              Foundation awareness week.

Chapter 3 -   I'm doing everything right but   37
              I still feel ill.

Chapter 4 -   Getting the message heard,   53
              an impossible task?

Chapter 5 -   How do I tell others exactly   61
              how this feels?

Chapter 6 -   MS versus APS   67

Chapter 7 -   2003 was not a good year for me!   75

Chapter 8 -   Depression and Anxiety   95

Chapter 9 -   Wendy- The reason we should   107
              all fight for the correct treatment

Chapter 10 - So what's new?   113

Chapter 11 - Internet sites   119

Introduction

After writing Sticky Blood Explained, my first book, I became increasingly frustrated about the things I felt I'd missed out.

Learning about APS is very much an ongoing experience and by the time my first book was published I had lots more going on in my head. It seems to me that as time goes by, I seem to have more and more questions about Hughes Syndrome. By each appointment with Dr Hughes I have so many questions I want to ask it is a wonder that I remember my own health issues!

I am learning that nothing about this illness is "black and white". I have been outspoken when trying to help people on the internet support groups, thinking I knew everything at times, only to be pulled back down to earth by someone who has "been there" and doesn't fit the text book.

I do feel that this is my huge advantage, I have contact with the other patients and I hear all their grumbles on a day to day basis. Hughes Syndrome is not really a case of "put them on the warfarin and all will be fine"; there are ongoing problems and people who do not respond as they should, to treatment.

There is so much yet to be done with this illness. There are so many unanswered questions. There needs to be a lot more research before we can understand fully what is happening in our complicated bodies.

I hope that for those who read my first book this one fills in a few gaps. I don't doubt that by the time this one is published there will be more questions buzzing around my head! It seems that with an illness as new as this one (though 20 years is hardly that new!) there will always be new developments to keep up with and more to find out.

One thing you can be certain of, as I find out more, I will pass that on to you!

Chapter 1
Those endless tests and How to survive them

As I sat with a member of the support group I run, the above title came to me. She was waiting for a scan and was very apprehensive about both the test and the possible results. I tried my best to help but I really felt inadequate. As soon as I was back at home the research began in earnest. All of the tests I have described are often used to look for problems when you have Hughes Syndrome, though they are often used for other unrelated problems in people with other illnesses too.

I would hate anyone to read this chapter and be terrified. It is a point of reference for when you need a test, not a list of tests you will have. Most people have a few of the tests or you may have already had some of them. Don't imagine you will need more than a fraction of these performing on you. It all depends on how APS has affected you. I have tried to describe each test and what it involves. I have then tried to say what the doctor may be looking for. I have also talked with others about coping strategies. Most of the information about tests that I have given is based on real people's experiences, the Internet APS forums have been only too grateful to supply me with any piece of information that may help another patient in need. Tests may be a routine matter for medical staff but for the patient it is quite another matter. The fear of the unknown is very daunting and imaginations can run wild. Most medically trained people would agree that people tend to be calmer if they know what they are letting themselves in for.

There seem to be more questions relating to tests and what to expect than any other subject on the forums. I have split up the tests. Firstly I will talk of general tests which may be done on lots of different parts of the body. Secondly I will talk of specific tests concerning specific parts of the body and tests in pregnancy. Lastly I have briefly mentioned some of the tests used to diagnose associated illnesses. I have already spoken about the diagnostic tests for APS so I won't be repeating myself on that score.

General Tests

Blood Tests many of us with Hughes Syndrome have trouble finding our veins when we need blood tests. I have one really good vein, which I always point out when I have blood taken. Sometimes I think if you have a good vein perhaps a tattoo that says, "draw blood here" and an arrow pointing to the spot would be a good idea! The best piece of advice is to insist on butterfly needles if you have difficulties giving blood. This is a needle, with a tube attached, which is much less likely to bruise you, or cause pain. Also you will find that a skilled phlebotomist can find veins that no one else can and a good one hardly ever leaves a bruise.

X-rays X rays are often used, by doctors, when looking for answers to our many problems. They are of course painless and few people have never had an X-ray. It is just a standard run of the mill test, which most people understand so I won't go into detail

Computerised Axial Tomographic (CT or CAT) Scan this test uses X- rays to generate an image of a body part. The test is completely painless. It involves lying on a very hard bed for a few minutes whilst the machine scans whichever body part the doctors are looking at. The machine resembles a huge white doughnut and the body part being looked at is put inside the doughnut. It is not at all claustrophobic, as the hole in the centre of the ring shape is large and fairly shallow in depth. The worst part is that you have to stay still, (especially if you feel a bit dizzy). It seems as soon as you are told to stay still you really want to move. This is an easy test really and certainly absolutely nothing to worry about

CT Scan with contrast this is a CT scan just as above except that a dye in introduced through a vein. My friend told me that this is the weirdest feeling. In her words "you can actually feel it moving through your body, it's a feeling of warmth and goes through you, ending in the groin area and then you have the sensation that you are peeing in your pants!" "Once I actually had to look because it felt so much like it! The technicians said it's just a side effect and everyone does the same thing."
This test just shows the blood vessels more clearly than a standard CT scan.

Magnetic Resonance Imaging scan (MRI) for this test the patient is placed into a magnetic field. Bursts of magnetic energy are used which build up a very detailed picture of the affected body part. MRI gives very accurate images, which may show problems that could not be detected by other tests.
MRI is one test that few enjoy. It is rather claustrophobic as it is like going into a narrow tunnel. You lay on a hard table and the part being scanned needs to go inside the tunnel. The bed moves so all that is needed is for you to lie very still. There is a mirror above your head (if your head is the part

being scanned). This is so you can see the outside world is still there. You are given a panic button to press if you really can't bear to be inside the scanner. You can usually hear the person, who is doing the scanning and they may ask if you are still OK between scans. There is a noise rather like a jack- hammer going off. You are usually given headphones but this only muffles the sound a little. I have a few quotes from those who have had MRI scans.

"I guess the best advice I can offer re MRI scans is to make full use of the little mirror above your head. Because it is tilted, you can see outside the scanner. You feel a bit less claustrophobic and reassured that outside is not far away. If you feel really panicked, a friend of mine was actually given a sedative so perhaps that is an option."

"I have a friend who was taught a technique for stress management. She was told to actually have a specific memory or thought to go to when she feels herself pulled toward negative thoughts. For her it was a waterfall, with the sound of the cascade, and with her dog by her side. It works."

"Much as I wanted to press the panic button I resisted, I kept thinking, no I will only have to do this again, not much longer, stay calm. Its just mind over matter."

"I can't see what the fuss about MRI scans is. I just closed my eyes and relaxed. All I had to do was stay still; there is no pain. In fact I almost fell asleep."

As you can see different people have different ideas. I think the main thing is to remember, it may be noisy and a small space but it doesn't hurt and it will soon be over.

Doppler Ultrasound this involves a hand held device called a transducer, which sends sound waves through whatever is being scanned. A Doppler ultrasound is painless. It involves some jelly being put on the body part and the transducer

being run over it. This produces a moving image as the waves travel through tissues and reflect back. The results are seen on a screen, which you can usually see if you wish.
No one usually has any problems or fears with this type of test.

Tests for Stroke
Radioactive Angiography radioactive compounds are injected into an arm and the blood stream carries them to the head. As the radioactive compound circulates it gives out bursts of radiation. This can be detected and forms an image of the brain. This can show doctors whether parts of the brain have been deprived of blood and are therefore damaged. The only discomfort is the initial injection. You may feel a warm, flushed feeling

Electroencephalogram (ECG) Electrodes are placed on your scalp for this test. These electrodes detect electrical activity in the brain and send it back to a machine, which records them on paper. By observing these impulses underlying problems in the brain can be detected. This test is painless and you will only have to stay still for a very short time.

Evoked Response Test these tests provide a measurement of how well your brain is processing and reacting to stimuli of different sorts. These can be visual images, sounds or stimulation of a nerve in the arm or leg. Depending on the responses you give, the doctor can tell where any possible damage to the brain may be. This may seem at times like a childish game, but serious problems can be detected in this way.

Carotid Phonoangiography A microphone, which is very sensitive, is placed on your neck to record sounds in the carotid artery. The carotid arteries are the main blood supply to the brain so obviously blockages here are very serious. In normal arteries the blood flow is smooth and controlled, but in arteries which are partly blocked the blood flow is turbulent (like water in a river when there are lots of bends in it). If this turbulence is heard more tests will be needed. This is a painless test.

Digital Subtraction Angiography For this test a catheter is introduced through an artery in the groin. You remain conscious but may be given a mild sedative to help you relax. The catheter is threaded through the blood vessels and watched on a screen. When the catheter reaches the site of the suspected blockage a dye is introduced through the catheter and outlines the blood vessels. The whole thing can be seen on a screen. The groin area is numbed with a local anaesthetic so that you feel nothing. As with other procedures involving dye you will feel a warm flushed feeling. When the catheter is removed pressure is applied to the puncture site until it seals. No stitches are needed but you will have to lie in bed for a few hours to be sure the site has sealed properly. You will have some bruising but it is really not too bad usually. An X ray machine quickly takes pictures of the head and neck when the dye reaches those vessels and the images let doctors identify and localise the site of the stroke.

Heart Tests
Cardiac Catheterisation this is exactly as described above for Digital Subtraction Angiography except that the doctors take images of the blood vessels around the heart. This test is really nothing to worry about and some people even find the whole experience fascinating. This can find blockages in the Coronary arteries. Sometimes these blockages are treated, by inserting a balloon into the catheter and inflating it at the

site of the blockage. The warm feeling as described so well by my friend in the section "CT scan with contrast" is the most alarming part of the whole thing. Most people do find that strange but a little amusing as well.

Treadmill Test (Stress Test) this involves stripping to the waist to have electrodes attached to your chest. You can then put your T- shirt on top. (I will admit it, I had visions of running topless which is not funny if you have a large chest). (OK perhaps it is funny.) You are then put onto a treadmill and as you are put through your paces, walking slowly and then quickly, then climbing a slope etc, a doctor checks the readout from the electrodes and checks your blood pressure. If you are unable to get to the end of the test it is a sign that you have a problem. If you reach the end and feel fine it is a good sign that your heart is probably fine. If at any time you feel unwell the test will be halted. Throughout the test a doctor carefully observes you.

Electrocardiogram (ECG) This test involves lying on a bed and having electrodes attached to your chest, (yes it does involve the dreaded topless bit girls), and to your feet. A paper record is made of your hearts electrical current and the whole test only takes a minute. This test can show that you have had a heart attack or sometimes, severe angina shows up on it.

Echocardiogram this is an ultrasound of the heart using sound waves. It is painless. A gel is applied to the chest and the hand held scanner is run over the skin. This shows the blood flow through the heart and shows how the heart is functioning. It also shows any area of damage to the heart muscle.

Holter Monitoring this is a continuous ECG recording of your heart as you go through your usual routine. It is usually worn for 24 hours. It is a small box, like a Walkman, attached by wires to patches on your chest under your clothes. You may be asked to write down the time of any strange symptoms whilst you are wearing the holter. This test assesses your heart condition.

Lung Tests
VQ Scan this is a test done in two parts. The first part involves a small amount of a radioactive drug being introduced into your arm. You will be told to sit in front of or lie beneath a camera, which takes pictures to show how the blood flows to your lung. Also a small amount of radioactive gas is given with an oxygen mask. About 12 hours later you will have a chest X-ray. As a friend of mine said " X rays showed hardly anything, but this test showed hundreds of clots in my lungs, and there was no discomfort at all from the test."

Blood Gases this test involves taking blood from an artery in your arm. The site can be anaesthetised, if you wish. There may be brief throbbing or cramping at the puncture site. Pressure will be applied to the puncture site for a few minutes after the test, to prevent bleeding. The test is used to evaluate lung problems or to determine how effective oxygen therapy is.

Lung Function Tests these are a series of tests to measure how well the lungs are working. Spirometry is performed by the patient breathing into a mouthpiece connected to a spirometer, which records the amount and rate of air breathed. You will be asked to breathe normally or exhale or inhale sharply.

Lung volume is measured in a couple of ways. The most accurate is a plesmythograph. You sit inside it (it is like a clear telephone box.) You then breathe in and out into a mouthpiece. Lung volume can also be measured by breathing a gas through a tube for a set amount of time. When the gas in the chamber, which is left at the end of the test is measured, an estimation of lung volume can be made.

Diffusion Capacity means that you breathe carbon monoxide for a very short time, even as short as one breath. The amount of carbon monoxide exhaled is measured and compared to that inhaled. This helps to estimate how quickly gas is travelling from the lungs into the bloodstream.

The tests can be unpleasant but not painful. There may be a clip on your nose and a tight mouthpiece to breathe through.

Tests for DVT

Venography this is the most accurate test for a deep vein thrombosis, but it can be uncomfortable and sometimes cause inflammation. Dye is injected into a large vein in your foot or ankle and an X-ray shows the location of any clots. Since venography is invasive and expensive it is more usual to use a Doppler scan as previously described. The Doppler is non-invasive and painless and can show clots usually quite well enough where they are most dangerous above the knee. Below the knee, Doppler is less effective and venography may be used.

Extra Tests in Pregnancy since APS pregnancies are considered high risk for both mother and baby, there are extra tests used. If you are receiving the correct care you will be closely monitored especially in the later stages of pregnancy. Regular ultrasounds should be done to check the baby's growth. Also special ultra sounds should be done to check the flow of blood through the placenta and the blood flow through the arteries in the area of the uterus. In the later stages of pregnancy a non- stress test should be done at regular intervals, which measures the baby's heart rate using two monitors on the mothers' abdomen. It makes a paper printout of the baby's heartbeats and measures the heart rate on a read out. This is done to monitor the baby's heart rate and looks for normal accelerations of the heart rate when the baby moves. Also special ultrasounds to measure the amount of amniotic fluid around the baby should be performed. All of these tests help doctors decide whether the baby is thriving and whether it is better to deliver early or leave well alone.

Tests for associated illnesses

Lupus In the main Lupus is diagnosed with blood tests and because of a collection of symptoms. Some of the blood tests usually done are called ANA, ESR, Rheumatoid factor, CBC, Renal and live profiles, Anti-dsDNA, and a few others.

Sjogrens The tests for Sjogrens include a Schirmer test, which is a piece of filter paper placed under the lower eyelid. This determines the amount of tears produced by your tear glands. It is not as uncomfortable as it sounds. Another test is called a slit lamp examination. This means a dye is dropped into the eye and then the eye is examined for signs of dryness or erosion. A salivary function test measures the amount of saliva in your mouth. There are blood tests that can be done but not everyone with Sjogrens will test positive. Other tests may include urine tests and chest X-rays. A lip biopsy is sometimes done, where a very small bit of your lip is cut away and examined.

Thyroid tests the main test is a blood test to measure various thyroid hormones in the blood and also to measure Thyroid

Stimulating Hormone, which is produced by the pituitary gland.

Apart from that you may have an ultrasound examination of your neck area to see if the Thyroid is enlarged. Sometimes a scan involving radioactive iodine is used (similar idea to other radioactive tests previously described in this chapter). These scans are painless and nothing to worry about.

General Strategies for coping with stressful times. A compassionate friend can be the best thing on earth if you are nervous. We can all benefit from a bit of "hand holding" and a few calming words of wisdom. If it helps you to relax take a friend or partner, (try to choose someone who will keep you calm rather than tell you tales of horror from things they have had done to them.)

Focus your mind on something happy or drift off in your mind to somewhere else. I mentioned one person's place, the waterfall. My "place" is on a sandy beach with waves crashing on the shore. As a mother of four teenagers I am pleased to report I am alone and in perfect peace. This is enough to make me relax, bliss, no heavy rock music blasting away.

Concentrate on one point in the room. Even if it is only a damp patch on the ceiling, staring at it may stop you from panicking.

Finally here's the one my friend used. Promise yourself a treat if you manage to get through the test without any problems. As she said, when she was a little girl, if she was good, she got a treat. Well why not? It's a darned good excuse I think.

Pass the chocolate!

Chapter 2

The very first Hughes Syndrome Foundation awareness week

In September 2002 from the 1st to the 7th was the first awareness week for this illness. I feel that in years to come this will be a landmark. A time when the illness began to properly emerge from being totally unknown to a well- known and understood illness.

The "Bridges of London" sponsored walk - After a seemingly endless build up for months before, the morning of September 1st started awareness week. It was a Sunday and a gloriously warm and sunny late summers day. My friend Sue and daughter Katie were with me in London. Today was the sponsored walk to raise funds for the Hughes Syndrome Foundation (HSF) and my friend and daughter were walking on my behalf. The walk was named the "Bridges of London", as the walkers would cross back and forth over every bridge between Tower Bridge and Westminster Bridge near to the hospital. The walk was to end at the Lupus clinic at St Thomas' hospital. All the 50 to 60 walkers met at Tower Hill tube station ready to walk over the first bridge, Tower Bridge. Both Dr Hughes and Dr Khamashta were there, looking somehow less comfortable than usual, when they are in their normal role tending the sick. They chatted to everyone and Dr Hughes seemed quite determined to be sure he spoke to everyone on that day, I don't think he left anyone out. I caught sight of him several times scanning the room, after the walk had ended, to be sure he had said hello to everyone he knew. There were nurses, and other staff from the clinics. People who worked for The Hughes Syndrome Foundation were there. Friends of people who were too ill to walk themselves. A few of the fitter patients walked as well. A few people had their dogs with them. Caroline handed out T-shirts to everyone and name badges.

After a few photos and some chat, at 11am they set off, walking in, groups of about 10 so as not to cause congestion on the footpaths. My friend Judi and I are both in the class of patient who dare not attempt to walk that far, angina is too unpredictable, and we didn't want to make ourselves ill and be a nuisance, so we got a taxi back to St Thomas' hospital. We were in charge of refreshments, so decided to go to a nearby supermarket to find beer, soft drinks and snacks. We set off on foot as it wasn't far, but to our dismay when we arrived we found there were no shopping trolleys and the staff in the shop were unhelpful to say the least. I was determined we wouldn't be beaten, so I asked a stunned lady at the front of the shop whether I could use her trolley. I tried my best to explain that we both had angina and this was all for a charity but she must have thought I was crazy. Once suitably loaded, the trolley was an unwieldy vehicle, but it would have been impossible for either of us to carry our shopping. We decided our only option was to steal the trolley to get the shopping back to St Thoms. Judi pushed whilst I pulled, the trolley had a mind of its own. The road back seemed far longer; crossing roads was an art, which we had perfected by the time we finished. We sat and had a rest, as both of us were terrified we would set off our angina. Judi and I had to giggle as we went along, it just seemed so ridiculous. Two large ladies pushing a trolley full of beer and crisps, and having to rest because they both had angina. Thank goodness we arrived at the hospital a little out of breath but OK. We sat on a wall and waited for the walkers, still laughing at what a silly thing we had done. We did feel quite proud that we had done it against all odds. Little things please you when you are used to being restricted by illness.

At about a quarter to one the first lady returned. Behind the leader came a few more, Katie and Sue amongst them, and gradually they all came, looking a little weary but as though they'd enjoyed it. After all, the sights of London were all along the route, there had been plenty of photo opportunities along the way. The drinks were the first priority as the day was warm. Judi and I hadn't done our trolley dash in vain. A wine merchant had supplied bottled water, wine and more beer and kindly stayed to serve it and our contribution, to the tired walkers. The whole day was fun and friendly. We all enjoyed the experience and raised lots of money for research, support and awareness of Hughes Syndrome. As the sun shone down, on that day, London seemed a great place to be, full of life and laughter, tinged with hope that we would make a difference.

The Children's Party - the next event for awareness week was to be a party in the Governors hall at St Thomas'. It was a party for some of the many children born due to the work of Dr Hughes and Dr Khamashta and their colleagues. The children's mothers had Hughes Syndrome and most had, had multiple miscarriages or still births prior to treatment. The party was attended by a few celebrities, mums and dads, the doctors, various helpers, and of course about 60 children. They had an entertainer and all the usual party food, and I'm sure the sight of them all together must have made Dr Hughes and Dr Khamashta feel very proud.

The event was filmed live by BBC television. They were filming a programme called City hospital at St Thomas hospital at that time and the party featured on that. First was an interview with Dr Hughes and a patient, talking about

Hughes Syndrome. The patient was a young woman; she described how she had lost the sight in one eye and was going blind in the other eye. She was referred to Dr Hughes when it was found she had the APS antibodies in her blood. Dr Hughes gave her Warfarin and once her blood was anti-coagulated her eyesight returned. She said it was almost immediate and you could sense the disbelief in the voice of the interviewer as they asked her about it. The young woman looked at Dr Hughes for confirmation that what she had said was true and they smiled at each other. This was yet another miracle of many, but what a difference to this woman's life. Then, there was an interview with some parents and a little boy with Dr Khamashta. The lady had, had many miscarriages and a still birth before having her miracle baby. I hope that if there were any women watching who felt, perhaps this was the cause of their miscarriages, rushed out and got tested as this lady urged them to do. There was also an interview with one of the patrons of the Hughes Syndrome Foundation, Triona Holden, a former BBC broadcaster. She did an excellent job of describing the illness to the stunned presenter who couldn't believe how little was known about this illness by anyone other than those involved with it. Anyone watching who was in the early stages of Hughes Syndrome and didn't realise that this could be the answer must have been thinking, "I wonder if that is what is wrong with me." Hopefully a few people asked their GPs to send them for the blood test.

The power of the media cannot be over emphasised. It is through the TV and newspapers that we learn about everything that happens in the world. It is only through endless bombardment that the message will get through. One article or one TV programme does not make something a household name, it is the constant talking and reporting of things which forces people to listen. We need the world to listen so that every new Hughes Syndrome patient gets the correct care in future. It is up to us, the patients to keep on trying.

The Patients Forum - I had looked forward to this forum for months. My husband was in London with me but he decided not to come to the actual forum. It was much better that he didn't as I was meeting with my friends who I had only spoken to on the Internet or by telephone before. I wanted to be a free spirit for that day so I could chat and wander, without feeling I must keep making sure he was OK. He is not keen to know any more than the basics of APS, so dragging him along would have been wrong for both of us. I also think that unless your partner is very interested in the illness it really isn't necessary to force feed them with the facts. I met up with Judi and Liz; a member of the local support group I run, outside the Lupus clinic at St Thomas' and we all set off to find the Governors Hall. I smiled because though Liz and Judi had never met before, they were chatting away non-stop. I think once you have something serious like APS to discuss the conversation starts and before you know where you are, people are your friends. We turned left at the wall plaque of Queen Elizabeth's head and looked out for the statue of Queen Victoria, whom Judi said, had a spaceship flying above her. I laughed when I saw it. It was a modern light fitting which looked completely out of place and yes it did look a bit like a spaceship. We wondered whether it was permanent or a temporary fixture. (I have since discovered it IS permanent! Oh dear!) In the corridor we met Sandra, another member of my support group with her daughter. Of course we arrived way too early and ended up going for a coffee and Liz and Judi just kept on chatting.
When we went back we were met at the door and handed our name badges and a badge with the HSF logo on it. We now

looked quite official. The room was panelled and very grand. I immediately spotted Michelle, who we all talked to on the Internet and we laughed about her husbands, sponsored beard shave for awareness week to take place that day. He just smiled if he was worried he didn't betray it.

We had a buffet lunch, which was lovely but I kept looking around and thinking surely she/he hasn't got Hughes Syndrome. There were so many faces I didn't know and apart from my little gang we really didn't talk very much at this stage. Another friend Sarah came in, it was funny but even though we had never met it seemed that we just knew each other instantly. We all filed into the Governors hall bit by bit, by then I had begun talking to a lady called Brigitte and my friends called me saying they had saved a seat. I made my excuses and left Brigitte, as my little gang were getting quite insistent that I should "get a move on!" I had to smile when I saw them all sat on the front row. I would have sat nearer to the back but I took my place there in between Michelle and her mum, with all my friends around me. I felt as if I had known them for a very long time and we had talked about so many things by e mail, that I guess we knew more about each other than many of our oldest friends knew.

Dr Hughes - Dr Hughes climbed onto the podium to speak. There were slides to illustrate his talk He went through all of the symptoms of Hughes Syndrome. As he did this Michelle's mother beside me was gasping and shaking her head from time to time. Now and then Michelle and her mum exchanged worried glances. I think a lot of it was hitting home with her and it was the first time she had heard the real seriousness of this illness. For a quiet and unassuming person Dr Hughes spoke very well, but there, he must have done this many, many times. I had only seen the quietly enthusiastic man in his consulting room, never on a stage.   I can't honestly say there was anything in his talk that I didn't already know about Hughes syndrome, but I could tell that others in the room were not as knowledgeable. They were shocked and surprised by what he was telling us. He told us one or two stories of people's experience with Hughes Syndrome, which really drove home some of the points he was making. I was really interested to hear about how he first realised that one of his patients had a blood- clotting problem, which was causing her problems. To hear from the man himself, about how he came to realise that this was a separate illness from Lupus in the early 1980's was so interesting, I felt privileged to sit and listen to a little piece of medical history.

He did a very complicated illustration, which I will never be able to remember, about Queen Anne having Antiphospholipid Syndrome, and how this led to American Independence! It was in there as light relief and we all laughed, we needed to laugh I suppose. Dr Hughes told us all about home testing your INR and why it cost the National Health Service far less if people had control of their own INR. One lady had 7 leg thromboses (DVT) in a year due to her swinging INR pattern. She was a determined sort and then persuaded her local supermarket to pay for a home- testing machine so she could test her own INR and adjust her dose of Warfarin, so preventing the swings in her INR. She had no further DVTs. Her DVTs had cost the National Health Service, in the region of £70,000. The machine cost £399. Not to mention the improvement in her health.

He then told us that we were all well educated in that room, we were the ones who shouted and knew how to fight our way to the front. He asked us "what about people who are not so well educated, or not so willing to speak up?" I could see he was telling us, we were just the tip of a very large iceberg, as we were the persistent ones who wanted answers and had the means to find them. We were the ones who dared to question doctors and fight for the right treatment. It made me wonder just how many more people are out there suffering and at risk through lack of awareness in the medical profession. He told us, it wasn't us that needed educating, it was the doctors. I know I said that I already knew most of what Dr Hughes was telling us, but I had always felt that perhaps in my book I had overstated the seriousness of APS and now I knew I hadn't. I had been afraid of upsetting people or frightening them but this talk made me see that what I had written had to be said. This talk uplifted me and made me feel that what I had done was right. I felt whatever happened I would do anything to help the cause of better awareness of Hughes Syndrome and its implications.

Dr Khamashta - Dr Khamashta sees mainly the patients who have had problems in pregnancy. He talked about the terrible pain and anguish women go through when they have miscarriage after miscarriage. Again I don't think there was anything he said that I hadn't found out about whilst researching to write this book, but his enthusiasm made you feel the facts. He was very enthusiastic throughout and I felt he seemed angrier than Dr Hughes about the injustice involved in this illness. (Though I doubt that Dr Hughes feels any less angry, it is just not as obvious). The two differing personalities showed. Dr Hughes was calm and quietly getting things done without betraying his feelings too much. Dr Khamashta had all his feelings there on show for everyone. I could empathise with that angry feeling that so many are suffering needlessly. I too felt angry when I thought of the undiagnosed out there unknowingly waiting for a disaster to befall them. If he was annoyed, I was as well and most of the room felt the same I'm sure.

Again we heard stories of real patients and their struggles. Dr Khamashta ended by talking about Dr Hughes and how much he deserves to have the honour of having this syndrome named after him. He told us how other doctors had doubted Dr Hughes, even thinking he was a fanatic, how Dr Hughes had set up the Lupus in pregnancy clinic. How he had carried on treating people and studying APS whatever anyone else tried to tell him. It became obvious that he idolises Dr Hughes and rightly so. I don't think there can have been a person in that room who didn't think Dr H was the bee's knees.

Question Time - once both doctors had done their talk it was time for questions from the audience. I thought for a dreadful moment that no one was going to speak so I flung my arm in the air before I had time to think better of it. I asked about the patient's theory on micro clots, which I mentioned in my chapter about feeling ill even though you are doing everything correctly. I think perhaps my question was a bit before its time but Dr Khamashta agreed that this theory was possible and in time more accurate scans might prove the theory. He also added that Warfarin was not to treat headaches primarily but to prevent blood clots. He said that the addition of aspirin often helped. Dr Hughes looked a little surprised at my question as he probably remembered that I had told him I had stopped taking aspirin and that I was feeling very well only a month earlier. I was asking on behalf of others really, not myself and my question was one thing that I really wanted to know for my book.

The floodgates then opened and lots of people wanted to ask questions and relate their stories. Most people's questions were the sort that my book could have answered, in other words the sort of questions that I, and other members of the Internet APS forum, had already asked each other. Every time there is a batch of new members the same old questions get asked over and over, which was my motivation for writing about this illness. Two stories stick in my mind. One was a woman who was there with her husband. She described many of the symptoms of APS, told us she had, had blood clots and she did test positive for the antibodies. She was not taking any anticoagulants however. When she said she had suffered a minor fit on the train there was a gasp from some of the audience. Dr Khamashta sounded angry and asked her why she wasn't taking Warfarin? She answered that her doctor had taken her off Warfarin, as it was such a "nasty" drug. Dr Hughes then spoke and told her she must start taking Warfarin immediately and he would speak to her doctor. He said she was sitting on top of a volcano waiting for it to explode unless her blood was properly anticoagulated. Moments after this a young man stood up and told us the story of his wife, it was the old familiar story of doctors not taking her seriously, so I suppose most of us were not taking every word in. We had heard a few stories of people's hell prior to diagnosis by now and we'd all been there ourselves. Then he dropped the bombshell; his wife was dead due to APS and a lack of correct treatment. There was a hush and you could feel the atmosphere change in the room. I felt close to tears and looked at my friends, between us we had, survived strokes, a heart attack, and a pulmonary embolism all either a few years before or after our 40th birthday. We were all damaged in some way, but we were alive and so easily it could have been us who died instead. I think every survivor in that room was thinking, "there but for the grace of god go I." I felt so sorry for the woman who had spoken earlier, I did think "well I know she will seek help now." Indeed I spoke to her and her husband after the talk and I was confident that they would get her "sorted out" as fast as they could. What luck that they decided to come to the forum. What a terrible shame that luck had to come into it.

By now I was on the edge of my seat longing to ask people "Why don't we all get together and do something, there are enough of us here." But I never got the chance again as everyone had things to ask and I figured their need was greater than mine was. After the questions had ended Dr Hughes invited us to go through for a cup of tea, but people queued to talk to both doctors. Both of the doctors patiently listened and advised everyone who wanted their help. When I think of how busy those two men must be and all the people needing their help, I feel I will never again say I'm too busy. They don't seem to be too busy for anyone.

The beard shaving. - Michelle's husband Howard, bravely volunteered his face to Dr Hughes for shaving. He had a full beard and had said he would have it shaved off to raise money for the foundation. Well Dr Hughes is very good when it comes to medical matters, but I think the barbers of London are quite safe if he is their competition. Dr Khamashta also had a try, but in the end the poor man went off to do the deed himself. When he returned he was unrecognisable, but he raised a nice amount for the Foundation and as Michelle said it would soon grow back. Well done Howard!

Tea and lots of chat - Well after we had all been in that room together it no longer mattered whether we knew each other, we were all chatting and swapping stories. It felt like being part of a very large family, we all had something in common and we all knew how it felt. There is nothing to beat looking into a friend's eyes, as you tell them about your headache or whatever, and seeing the look of recognition and empathy, instead of the look of indifference or boredom anyone else might give you. I really felt that something had happened that was significant that day. We were the pilgrims and now we needed to spread the gospel. Judi and I walked together for a while after it all ended and when we parted I think we both felt strange. We had shared so much in that week and now we were going back to e- mails. We promised to keep in touch and meet up again. Of course we have and probably always will now.

I do get the feeling at times that I am obsessed with raising awareness of Hughes Syndrome. After attending the forum I was buzzing with all the things that were said for a week or more. I try very hard to maintain a balance between fighting the fight and normal day to day living. Saying, "I'm all right now, so let the rest get on with it" isn't my way, I can't do that, I wish I could sometimes. It's not about being better than other people or anything grand or clever, it is just that some of us can't say no, and can't turn our back on others, as much as we may want to at times. Not getting involved, just isn't an option, I am involved, but my normal living has to come first and I am careful to remember that. Still I find it impossible to keep my head down and say nothing when I feel passionately about something. A doctor once told me to keep my head below the parapet and not get into the firing line. It's advice I've found impossible to take.

On this day, at the forum, I had met others who felt the same way about Hughes Syndrome as I did, and it felt wonderful. The battle to get more recognition and understanding for this condition has to go on so that one day every doctor in the world will know what Hughes Syndrome means.

Chapter 3
I'm doing everything right but I still feel ill.

Oh dear, the trouble with the miracle of Warfarin is that it isn't a cure. If it were a cure we would all be able to shut up as we would be back to normal, and this book wouldn't be needed at all. All that Warfarin can do is treat the problem of sticky blood by thinning it. The root cause, whatever that may be, is still there.

The illness, Hughes Syndrome is incurable and is still there even when all available treatment is being used to the full. Treatment can only relieve some of the problems, which are caused by it, such as blood clots. It is a bit like when you have a cold, you take cough medicine to relieve your cough but as soon as you stop taking the medicine the cough returns. Warfarin helps with the symptoms, saves you from serious clotting, but won't cure your illness. That said, there are many people who feel completely fine once they are well controlled on the Warfarin regime. It is really a question of how lucky you are and how soon you were diagnosed.

Micro clots? - I have noticed by talking to others. with APS on the Internet that the vast majority of people still have ups and downs. I think everyone would say they are miles better than they were before their blood was thinned but there may still be bad days even after treatment One explanation for this is a theory that a few of us on the internet forums worked out. Perhaps anticoagulation with Warfarin or whatever protects us from the big nasty clots, that can cause strokes, DVT, and heart attacks, but there are still tiny "micro" clots floating about in our blood. These would be too small to seriously clog any major blood vessels but perhaps now and then they affect smaller vessels and cause headaches, memory loss etc, on a smaller scale than before. It would make sense that from time to time we would feel less well or have minor problems like pins and needles. I have asked Dr Hughes about this theory and he agreed it was possible. The trouble is that scanning techniques cannot yet pick up these "micro" clots so our theory will remain just that, a theory for now.

A "too low" - INR Another explanation for the way we can wax and wane with the various symptoms of APS despite treatment, is that our INR is not properly controlled. When feeling unwell I always check my INR and very often it has slipped a little lower than it should be for me. This is easily remedied with a small change to the warfarin and rechecking in a few days. Of course a home testing device is necessary for this to work. If your blood is only being tested monthly at a clinic, there is a good chance your INR has gone up and down in between checks. We are often very INR sensitive the difference between an INR of 2.6 and an INR of 3.5 can be a huge thumping headache that refuses to budge, gets in bed with you and is still there in the morning. Other problems such as concentration or memory loss can wax and wane depending on where your INR is on that day as well. This can sometimes be remedied by taking an aspirin or another anti platelet drug as well as Warfarin. Usually doctors don't recommend that both drugs be taken together but in our case it may be needed. Aspirin causes the platelets to be less sticky and less likely to stick together. For some reason not yet understood (but perhaps the patients forum micro clots theory fits), just the addition of aspirin or another anti platelet drug can stop the headaches and brain fog.

If the INR is fine and in your target range
In some of us our INR can be completely fine and yet still we have headaches, memory loss and other APS related problems. As I have said before not on the scale they were before but bad enough to really make you feel ill and fed up. It may be that your target INR is not high enough and you need to experiment with a slightly higher INR to see if you feel better. This is OK to try so long as you aim to stay below 4. Above 4 you won't just bleed to death, people get far higher by mistake and live to tell the tale, but there is a higher risk of bleeding once you get over that figure. I have often been far higher and had nothing terrible happen but it's not sensible to do this on purpose. I do know people whose target range is above 4, but this must only be because your APS doctor has advised it, not on a whim. If your INR is as high as you can reasonably try and you still have terrible symptoms then the addition of aspirin or Plavix can make a huge difference.

I have an example from my own experience. I was taken off aspirin when my stomach started to complain. At first I felt fine and had no problems. A month or two later I developed a long lasting headache which went on for a fortnight. It was a fuzzy, muzzy feeling and I really could not think straight. When asked a question I started to really struggle to answer. I felt exhausted and as though my mind was not my own. I took my tablets in the wrong order one day; I took my Warfarin at breakfast and was amazed in the evening to find my other distinctly different tablets waiting for me! (One was even a purple torpedo shaped tablet so how I managed to confuse the two piles of tablets I have no idea.) I felt sick that I could do such a stupid thing, it should have been obvious to me that the pile of 9 tablets was for the morning and the pile of 4 were for the evening, I had been doing it correctly for years now. I checked my INR and it was perfect. I was confused, was I going crazy?

Then, I remembered that Dr Hughes had told me on my last consultation that if my headaches and confusion returned, it was probably because I had stopped taking aspirin. At the time I felt so well that I doubted that I would have a return of the headaches and dismissed what he had told me. He said if my headaches were to come back, I was to ask my GP to give me Plavix as a replacement for aspirin. He explained that, Plavix doesn't affect the stomach but still makes platelets less sticky. Within days of starting Plavix, I felt better and the headaches stopped. If it hadn't happened to me I would have found it hard to believe.

My friend had a neuralgia type headache even though her INR was quite high. It was very severe and endless. On Dr Hughes advice, she has found that an injection of heparin in conjunction with warfarin just when she has the headache, works like a charm. Most doctors would think that rather risky but it works and she is fine. There is an awful lot more to be discovered as yet about Hughes Syndrome and why some things work and others don't. It is all far more complicated than we can possibly imagine. It may be many, many years before everything is understood about APS and its mechanisms. However if you are suffering then you must tell your doctor and work together to find a solution. It seems that there are sub sets of APS patients , some respond to aspirin, others to warfarin , some need a combination to keep symptoms under control.

As my confidence in my own instincts about my illness has increased I have started experimenting with my treatment. I have discovered that my INR needs to be somewhere close to 4 or just above for maximum relief. If my INR creeps up to around 5 I still feel fine though I start to bruise and that tells me to test my INR and reduce my dose of warfarin. I don't bleed excessively even at around an INR of 5.

If my INR drops to less than 3.5 my angina gets worse so I have started giving myself a 20mg heparin injection if my INR drops close to 3.

Sometimes my INR is fine but I get one of those terrible never ending headaches. I have found that even though aspirin doesn't agree with me I can tolerate a "one off" baby aspirin in addition to my warfarin and plavix. This works really well for me and nothing bad has happened as a result!

I tell Dr Hughes of my experiments and he agrees that its fine for me to try if I feel OK about being my own little research guinea pig!! I feel increasingly confident about trusting my own judgements and not worrying about bleeding too much.

This of course is all what suits me and my situation. Each of us needs different management of our illness and we need to work with our doctors to find out what helps us. I wouldn't suggest that anyone else does anything without discussing it with their doctor first as it could be very dangerous. I am willing to take a small chance by trying things out now and then but that's my choice and my goodness I wouldn't suggest anyone else did the same!

What about the other connected illnesses?
Not every ache and pain we have will be to do with Hughes Syndrome. Many of us have several diagnoses. If you have Lupus, the muscle aches and fatigue are probably due to Lupus rather than Hughes syndrome if your INR is fine. If you have Sjogrens, it too causes fatigue and aches and pains. Many of us seem to have arthritis of one sort or another, which needs to be treated rather than just "put up" with. Current thinking is that APS does not cause arthritis but I have observed from the internet forums that there seem to be a high proportion of us with arthritic problems. Perhaps

having APS means that we are more prone to developing arthritis as well. Whatever the cause, there is no need to "put up" with joint pain. If there is any damage being done to the joint then treatment is needed so don't just put it down as "one of those things".

Angina makes you feel ill at times and it may not be your sticky blood always to blame. The main things that are really likely to be down to APS are headaches and neurological symptoms such as tingling, numbness, or eye co-ordination.

It is vitally important that if you develop a new symptom you don't just assume it is caused by APS or some other connected illness you may have. When my mouth was constantly dry I assumed it was because of my Sjogrens and sucked sweets, chewed gum, drank loads of orange juice. It turned out that I had diabetes! I was making myself so much worse by sucking sweets and drinking juice! If you have a new symptom worrying you then see your GP and ask if they think it is another illness or just a new symptom of your old one. It may be something treatable as mine was.

Drugs galore

Many of us take lots of tablets for various conditions. For example I take warfarin and plavix for APS, two different types of nitrate for angina, a pill which reduces the acid in my stomach, a blood pressure tablet. Plus one known as a calcium channel blocker which supposedly helps Syndrome X. More recently diabetes medication has been added to the list. I know that many of you will have a list just as long or longer than mine. Much as I try not to think about it, all of these tablets have an effect on your body. Some slow you down, some block reactions in some way; they all have a list of side effects as long as your arm. It is reasonable to suppose that some of the "feeling ill" is down to swallowing a cocktail of drugs every day Without that cocktail, many of us would have died by now, others would be sat in a chair unable to do normal tasks. Really we have to put up with the side effects as not taking our medicine results in a far worse fate. I know its not fair, especially if you are young, but really we must remember that tablets are a wonderful thing if it means we can live a more normal life. There is always, a lot of research into how each separate medication may affect you but none on how the combination of many medications may make you feel. Your poor body has a lot to contend with so be patient with it.

Damage that occurred before you were treated

Most people, unless they were lucky and were tested early enough, had a major clotting incident which led to doctors testing them for APS. This means that most of us have had a stroke or a heart attack or lots of DVTs or TIAs. If you have had a stroke there are parts of your brain that will never work correctly again, a heart attack means an area of heart muscle has died, a DVT has caused damage to the blood supply in your legs, a pulmonary embolism leaves scarring in the lungs. Permanent damage of one sort or another has happened to lots of us due to blood clotting before treatment. Even if you haven't had a major "event" the effects of sticky blood flowing through your blood vessels for many years can leave some smaller scale long-term damage. This damage once it has happened will never be repaired, what is done, is done. How can we be sure that the headache and memory loss, isn't an after effect of the stroke we had a few years ago or the multiple TIA's we had prior to treatment? How can I know whether my angina is partly because my heart is damaged? It is very hard to tell.

That occasional chest pain you have may be due to the damage, caused by the pulmonary embolism you had last year, leg pain may be down to damage from your DVT. So some symptoms, which persist after your INR is fine, may be due to old damage, which cannot be repaired. Having said that, if something is really worrying you be sure to get it checked rather than just assuming its old damage. Let us hope that no one in the future gets damage that is permanent. With improved awareness, I hope doctor's test for and treat APS before a clot, when people first start to feel ill, not when the damage is already done.

The minority for whom warfarin is not enough
Sadly there are a small minority of people who seem to re clot even at relatively high INRs. The key here is "small minority" so don't think that you are in danger. If you are in that group however it is a frightening place to be. Unfortunately even the best APS doctors are stumped by this phenomenon. The best suggestions are as follows.

Try adding either aspirin or plavix to your warfarin

Try adding an anti malarial such as Plaquenil into the equation.

If all else fails the only other weapons to try are immune-suppressing drugs.

I do also know of some people who have been unable to get properly stabilised on warfarin and have been advised to use heparin long term. Those who have done this, that I know, have reported that they have done well but really if you are a "problem" patient a lot of your treatment for a while may be trial and error to find out what works the best for you. Long term heparin is not usually recommended because if the risk of osteoporosis and because of the way it has to be taken (by injection). However if a stroke is the alternative the benefits outweigh the risks.

I know that some people have trouble getting reliable INR readings. It is believed that this is connected with having a positive lupus anticoagulant test. Somehow the lupus anticoagulant prevents the test from working reliably. However I have a positive lupus anticoagulant and my INRs are fine and reliable. If you are one of the people who finds their home testing machine and the lab never agree, you have to decide with your doctor, which is correct. The home testing machines are very accurate and I trust mine 100% but if you have doubts perhaps you should stick with hospital testing.

There is also hope in the form of new drugs being developed. One of these is an oral heparin, which may be the answer to many people's problems, but it takes time for new drugs to be tested and evaluated, especially for APS patients.

It is very important to stress that warfarin therapy works for a vast majority of patients and is at present the treatment of choice recommended by experts in this illness.

We are aiming for improvement rather than a "cure"

All of that said, most of us still suffer many symptoms, which may have been improved by anticoagulation but not cured completely. As an example I still have some memory problems with short- term memory. I look blank so many times and get that look of disbelief from others when I don't have a clue about something that supposedly happened to me only a week ago! I spent ages trying to get hold of my dad by telephone because I was sure he went on holiday for a week and should be home. It turned out he went for a fortnight and had very clearly told me that. For some reason these things just won't sink into my brain and stay there! I still get pins and needles now and then. I have a habit of saying the wrong word or especially the wrong name even if the right name is in my head, the wrong one keeps coming out of my mouth! How frustrating it is when that happens, I have been known to lose my temper over that one! (Well my family bless 'em were falling about laughing at me, when I said a very strange alternative name from the depths of my brain! They kept screaming the right name at me, only for the wrong one to keep right on coming out of my mouth!) Fatigue is an enormous problem, which comes and goes but is ever present to some degree. I refuse to say tiredness because so many people say "Oh I get tired too, you want to try working the hours I work". Extreme fatigue is something else, its something you don't know unless you have it. Working long hours isn't tiring for us, we just can't do it at all!

On the positive side I have no headaches, I have perfect eyesight again, I have no leg cramps, so many symptoms that I had are a distant memory now (with my memory distant could really mean lost forever!) My angina is still present but is far more easily controlled and I haven't suffered from uncontrollable unstable angina, which used to land me in hospital, ever since my blood was thinned. That has to be counted as a huge improvement. I do still have stable and predictable angina which I can cope with.

I am lucky as I know others who don't get the degree of relief that I have. It's not that unusual to still have problems but at least you are safer from clots if you still take your warfarin. You do have to think very carefully about how ill you were before treatment to realise how much worse you would feel without it.

There is more to APS than anyone yet knows
Remember that although Hughes Syndrome was first described in 1983 it is still a relatively new illness. There is so very much that even the best doctors do not understand about why we are ill. It is known that APS affects the blood vessels as well as the blood platelets, perhaps that is causing problems for some of us? This would cause things such as vasculitis and spasms in the blood vessels. Who knows how many other things are affected? A more recent finding

suggests that a form of demyelination (antibodies attacking the myelin sheath, which surrounds nerves in the body) may be caused by APS in a proportion of patients. This would explain why some people seem to suffer from MS type symptoms even after treatment. MS is caused by demyelination.

If the demyelination is caused by sticky blood however it seems that thinning the blood helps and can stop further deterioration. There may be some degree of "crossover" between the two illnesses in some people? An atypical form of MS caused by Hughes Syndrome perhaps?

Doctors at St Thomas hospital have found all sorts of things from indigestion to high blood pressure to early morning stiffness can be related to sticky blood. If the arteries, or even one artery, to the kidneys is blocked by a clot or blood flow is slowed by "sticky" blood it will cause high blood pressure. If the blood supply to the gut is compromised by APS it can cause cramps and indigestion. In time it will be found that many, many other problems are caused by APS, blood is needed in every part of the body, if the supply is reduced it causes so many problems that almost anything is possible. Checking your INR regularly and keeping it above 3 at all times, may improve many health problems, which you hadn't connected to APS.

There is so much research ongoing and so much more that needs to be done that it will possibly be another 20 years before the illness is finally completely understood, even then I guess new things will keep coming up. We have to go with what is known now and keep up to date with all new developments. Joining the Hughes Foundation can be a way of keeping abreast of the latest news. The newsletters are interesting and members are kept informed of new developments. Also it may seem that fund raising is something that all charities harp on about but if we all made a small effort to raise a little money it would help to fund much needed research if not to help us then perhaps to help our children or grandchildren.

Stress
It is vital for anyone with a long term illness to avoid stress as much as possible. This is for two reasons, too much stress can affect how you think and how you actually feel. It is very important to only do as much work as you can comfortably manage. If you push yourself over and over again, sooner or later you will become ill. Pace yourself and if you need to cut working hours or find a less stressful job then do it. Your life may have to change in order for you to feel fitter. I know how ill I feel when I've "over done" things, taking life easy isn't a crime if it means you have energy to enjoy yourself as well as work.
If you have a stressful event coming up such as moving house or a divorce, be sure to ask for help if you need it. Try to talk to someone if it's emotional stuff you need help with. If it's just brute force and physical help you need then organise help. Be aware that you may feel extra weary for a while and try to organise your life to build a few easy days in. Always remember that there will be another day when you can finish things off and rest when you need to. Try to do jobs in stages rather than pushing yourself to do it all in a day. Prioritise and leave less urgent things for another day. You may find that you can work all morning and then you collapse in a heap by lunch. If that's you then go with the flow and rest after lunch for as long as it takes.
 We all realise that physical stress can make us ill, but emotional stress can be far worse to deal with and can make you just as ill as having too much work to do!
I have learnt from bitter experience to try to avoid upsetting experiences. At times this is impossible but at least if you

know that upset will probably make you feel ill, you can be kind to yourself until you recover.

I sat up all night with an elderly relative as they died this year. It was the first time I'd seen someone die and the experience affected me deeply for a while. I was exhausted and ill for two weeks following her death although I did my best to keep going I fell asleep every afternoon and ached all over. My angina got worse and I generally felt unwell.

Even as I sat with her that night I was thinking "I bet I'll pay for this". It was a job I felt I had to do however so the two weeks following were justified. However do think carefully about taking on duties that may exhaust you physically or mentally as we are more fragile and it takes longer for us to bounce back after these traumas.

Don't "grin and bear it!"

For a long time I put up with someone who continually upset me, doing things that really hurt my feelings for no apparent reason. I think I got a little depressed for a few days after a particularly nasty telephone call, which served no purpose other than upsetting me. After a while I suddenly realised that my family, who love me, are far more important to me than this person. I had been forgetting my tablets and not looking after myself so well as usual, due to one unkind person's insensitivity. It dawned on me that this was a selfish and indulgent way for me to behave. I needed to put those important to me first and stay well for their sake. If I let one cruel person get me down and make me ill, my loved ones would have to pick up the pieces. I made the decision to no longer have contact with the person who caused me to be so sad. I just very calmly explained in a letter that I was too ill to deal with this sort of upset and wanted no more contact. This lifted a weight from my shoulders and I felt instantly happier and fitter than I had for a long time.

It is a shame to have to cut people out of your life but priorities change when you don't feel well over the long term.

I think that when you have an illness to live with, it is enough just to get yourself through each day. You really don't need anyone dragging you down or being negative. My advice would be to lose anyone like that from your life, you really don't need them. Concentrate on the people who are supportive and care about you, stop worrying about anyone else. It is far better to annoy someone who you find upsetting by being honest and straight about how they make you feel, than to put up with them and become ill with the effort. Just trying to be nice to someone when you really don't mean it, can be a strain. If people care about you they may try to change once you tell them how you feel, if they don't, then realise they aren't worth your effort any more. Put yourself first for your own and your loved ones sake.

Be Realistic

You need to try to be realistic, it is unlikely that you will ever be the fit person you used to be. Only very lucky people have that sort of miracle. You will most likely be ill from time to time and working full time may be a problem. However you can still do what is within your capabilities and be useful without exhausting yourself trying to be "normal". Indeed I think the acceptance that you have a long term incurable illness that can and will change your life can do more to improve your health than any number of tablets. Giving in and accepting change rather than fighting to stay "normal" can make all the difference to how you view your symptoms. Acceptance is the most important thing for your mental and physical health.

Also although of course it is a good idea to take the advice of health professionals, remember you are human! You have a life to live and though chocolate biscuits are not recommended, they can make life more enjoyable! Yes drinking is bad for you but once in a while I live dangerously and have one or two more than I should, just for the hell of it! If you do every single thing that the "experts" tell you to do you will still have APS, you may not live any longer by denying yourself things. Be sensible most of the time but don't overdo it and make your life miserable by always being good, go on be naughty now and then!

So Folks to sum it up.
To end this chapter which has been mainly a case of pointing out facts which we are inclined to forget, here is a bit of wisdom from my husbands elderly aunt Dora who had diabetes for more than 60 years. On a visit I complained that my angina was back and I had thought it had gone. She said " My dear, if you have an illness like this, you cannot be well all the time. It has to come back now and then to let you know it is still there. If it never came back again you wouldn't be ill, you would be cured!" That is very simple but oh so true.

Chapter 4
Getting the message heard, an impossible task?

It is a daily task for me, one that invades my life constantly, I am forever dreaming up ways to make people listen, in particular I long for doctors to listen to me. I dream of a room full of doctors listening to my every word as I explain exactly what Hughes Syndrome involves!

I foolishly and naively thought that an illness, which is as devastating as this one can be would be headline news. I thought that surely if I just told all the newspapers they would want the story of how so many people can be helped. I soon found out that it was like banging your head against a brick wall.

I also discovered that one story can make a difference but only a small difference. It needs many stories and endless media coverage before an illness becomes a household name.

Once I thought my book would make people take notice of me. No, sadly that is not enough. It takes more than one book written by a mere patient (never mind that I actually live with the illness I am merely a lay person), to make other doctors listen to their patients.

Recently a member of my support group (whom I found by getting myself in a local newspaper talking about my book) was in despair. She had the results of her blood tests from 1988, when she was diagnosed with lupus, she had been looking at them because she had been so ill recently and had read my book. She also remembered a doctor back in 1988 telling her she had sticky blood and telling her to take aspirin which she had done ever since. She had a short time taking warfarin after a blood clot but was told to stop taking it by a so- called "expert".

She had since had many TIAs, which had recently been confirmed by a scan. She had all the classic symptoms of Hughes Syndrome. The blood tests from 1988 clearly showed an extremely high IgG anticardiolipin result.

She begged a doctor to re test her after reading my first book. Finally she convinced him, despite having been told by her lupus specialist (the "expert" above) that there was no point as her lupus anticoagulant was negative. He told her that the TIAs were caused by high blood cholesterol!

She was in despair as she could see what was staring her in the face, she had Hughes Syndrome and needed treatment with warfarin as the aspirin she had been taking was obviously not enough.

Trying to get a doctor to listen to you when you are a mere patient is a nightmare at times! Some doctors hate their patients to have an opinion or to have read up about their illness. Some seem to think you are undermining them or trying to tell them their job. She had been told to stop looking back to her past tests and stop reading so much about her illness! How many of us would be dead if we listened to that sort of advice and how was she supposed to forget all of this when she was having TIAs and feeling so ill?

I am happy to report she has eventually been listened to. The second anticardiolipin test she begged for was positive, as she knew it would be. That and her scan results terrified her lupus specialist so much that he arranged for her to have an immediate re test to check again her levels of anticardiolipin antibodies and also see another doctor about restarting warfarin therapy.

I was so happy for her that I wanted to cry. She could hardly believe that she had finally managed to convince doctors to treat her Hughes Syndrome. I think it was only that the specialist was afraid that she would have a full- blown stroke and he would get the blame that finally did the trick. What a shame she had to endure the terror of knowing what could happen to her and feel as though, apart from me, no one else could see the danger she was in. We were so helpless to get her the help we knew she needed, it was like every road ended in a dead end. The supposed "expert" wouldn't listen to sensible arguments as he was too arrogant to take the views of his patient seriously. How frightening it is to be trapped like this.

At times like this even your family can be unsympathetic, they often just want you to do what the doctor says, even if you know that its wrong. Even in the sceptical times we live in, most people still believe doctors rather than people who actually have the illness. It is a horrific situation to find yourself in when you can see so clearly what is needed and yet no one will listen.

This was not the end of the story regarding the doctor who wouldn't listen to my support group member and left her without warfarin and close to having a stroke. Soon afterwards I became involved with a man whose sister in law had seen the same arrogant doctor. He had taken her off warfarin despite it clearly stating in her records that it was a life long treatment. This made her very ill and to cut a long story short she ended up having such poor circulation in her legs that they both had to be amputated and had probable catastrophic APS into the bargain. If warfarin had not been withdrawn this would have been unlikely to have happened to her. Whatever she decides to do, no one can give this young woman her legs back. It is scandalous!

My worry is that these are just two cases out of the many patients he sees. This one doctor is causing havoc in the lives of his APS patients because he isn't up to date with current research. This type of, non-treatment MUST end. Doctors must listen and learn now, people must be dying and it must end!

I have a great GP called John Parry who works with me on my project to stay well! I still had to suffer two years of being undiagnosed despite his best efforts. Once diagnosed I still had to find out what was the correct treatment by myself, (he had never heard of Hughes Syndrome or anticardiolipin antibodies at that time, he was not the only one). Thank goodness I have him on my side, with an open mind, ready to take me very seriously, even long before I had a heart attack to "prove" I was ill. Knowing he is there and ready to listen when I am ill relieves the terrible anxiety we all know so well. I know that whatever life throws at me in the way of illness he will listen and try to help me. He treats me as his equal as do all the good doctors I have seen. Without knowing he is there if I need him I really don't think I could cope with the uncertainty of my life. Listening to their patient is the most wonderful skill a doctor can have, listening carefully can provide all the answers. If only all doctors would just listen to their patients. That is often not the case, time and time again I hear terrible desperate tales of people's disastrous consultations with dismissive doctors who wouldn't listen to their concerns. That is why support as well as awareness is needed, without my support and encouragement my support group member might have given up and not had the courage to fight until she was heard at last. . I really feel like screaming to her doctor "stop talking and listen to what I say, I am trying to tell you things that you need to know". Sadly I doubt he would listen.

Please if you are a doctor don't think I am being unkind about the profession, I know some very wonderful doctors, I owe my life to some of them. Just please try to imagine having an invisible illness that makes you feel so ill you feel dying might be an easy way out at times. When tests for various illnesses turn out to be negative our family rejoices. They don't realise that when you feel very ill negative tests are awful. All you long for is to test positive for something, anything, just so you have a reason for feeling so ill. Eventually though, you have a positive test for anticardiolipin antibodies and /or lupus anticoagulant.

Next, imagine going for help to a doctor who is meant to be your saviour, you look forward to seeing them for weeks and pray they will know of a way to help you. You feel that here is the only person who can get you out of this mess, but then you are told either, they don't know what is wrong with you, or you are depressed, or that it is down to your age! (I had all of these things said to me at some stage prior to diagnosis and as for the age part, I was 36 and had no friends suffering as I was because of their age!) They may even say (and this is one that was said to me) "well you look very well so I think it is safe to presume you are well!"

 Then, what is far worse, imagine you have read extensively about your illness and discovered your treatment is incorrect and could endanger your life. You rush back to your doctor, full of fear for your life, only to be told to "stop reading so much, take away all that nonsense you have printed from the internet" and come away feeling desperate and afraid. Where do you now turn?

The answer is you keep asking for another doctor until you find one who will help. I know people who have gone through many, many doctors getting more and more anxious and stressed each time.

Why do we need to go through all of this, when the answer is so obvious to all of us who read a little about Hughes Syndrome? If we can find out what we need to do and we have NO medical knowledge why can't doctors also read a little? I know the job is a hectic one but if you have a patient who knows what is wrong and what needs to be done surely it warrants a little quick research on the internet at the very least? Can you try to credit people with having enough sense to work things out for themselves and at least check out what they try to tell you? I know there must be any number of people thrusting information at you about this or that illness, which you are sure they don't have, but please don't dismiss everyone out of hand.

It is a frustrating situation and a dangerous one to know what needs to be done and have no way of convincing doctors that you are right.

This awful problem keeps me keen to get the word out there. It's a constant battle and one I will never give up while there are people in this nightmare place, this limbo of waiting to have a serious blood clot in order for anyone to take you seriously.

The only answer is that everyone with the will to try must keep pushing the message about Hughes Syndrome.

I send my book out to doctors free of charge whenever I find one that will listen a little. I also send Dr Hughes book if they are more likely to listen to him. The Hughes Syndrome Foundation produced a special booklet aimed at doctors, which I intend to send to a few. I get in any newspaper or magazine that will have me (mostly local but I have plans!) I encourage all those people in limbo to never give up but keep plugging away until they get the help they need. If I ever get the chance to go on the TV you can bet I'll be there! I don't crave the limelight but I do see that if I don't push the message in as many ways as I can, I won't make the difference I want so much.

If the reader has any feelings about shouting Hughes Syndrome from the rooftops then please pester every newspaper and magazine you can. Don't hide your light, shine bright and show those still in the dark tunnel of despair that there is a great deal of hope. Join the Hughes Syndrome

Foundation, ask how you can help to spread the word. Now I am starting to sound evangelical about it but it is so important that I suppose that is how it makes me feel.

My goodness I hate having my photograph taken, I freeze in front of a camera! Still I overcome that minor detail when it helps to spread the word about APS, and tell myself it's not about what I look like, it's about the greater good!

I'm sure the rest of you out there are far more photogenic than I am. Anyway, if you feel strongly and passionately about spreading the word, then get out there and make a start. Hughes Syndrome needs everyone to talk about it to become well known. Stick posters up, hand out booklets and try anything that will gain a little publicity, you may save someone's life. I keep smiling to myself as I write, as I do realise I sound as though I am recruiting people to some weird Hughes Syndrome cult, but it is a serious business really.

There is no more wonderful feeling than knowing that through your actions you have saved someone else from suffering.

Chapter 5
How do I tell others exactly how this feels?

This is a never- ending problem. A fit person has no conception of how it feels to have a long term disability or illness. It is a very difficult thing for them to understand that though you may look well you may feel very ill. Hughes Syndrome is one of those "invisible" illnesses for the majority of the time. People understand being unable to walk at all, but not being too tired to walk very far, "surely if you can walk 50 yards you can walk 50 more?" They can see how dreadful it is to have an illness like Alzheimers but not how more minor short term memory loss can be devastating as well. They say "don't be silly, you must remember, you weren't listening to me." Sometimes they seem to think that if the information was important you must remember it, not realising that any information can be forgotten. Whether something was important or not makes no difference to whether you can remember it!

People understand if your balance is so bad, you cannot stand and need a wheelchair but not how it is to live with ongoing vague dizziness every day, they may say "pull yourself together, perhaps your ears need syringing, I often feel a bit dizzy!" People may understand arthritis if the joints look swollen or sore but try explaining muscle pain or stiff joints, most glaze over! The main trouble when trying to explain what life is like for us, is not the big serious problems, like strokes and heart attacks, people understand that.

It is the little everyday trials, or the endless fatigue that wears you down that they don't understand. Fatigue is not the same as tiredness. Feeling tired is normal after a busy day or a lack of sleep, or too many late nights. Fatigue means being unable to summon the energy to do normal everyday tasks like washing the floor or peeling the potatoes without endless rests or doing things in stages. It is overwhelming and very distressing. You can feel this way even though you have had a wonderful nights sleep and done nothing else all day. It is like a wave washing over you that takes over your body. How we long to just get on with life and never need to worry about when our energy will suddenly run out.

On top of this there is the constant anxiety eating away at your confidence. What if I have another clot? What if I start bleeding and it won't stop? Who will help me if I get ill again? There is a gap between the wonderful specialist who understands APS and your GP who knows only what you have told him. You can't get hold of the expert and your GP is reluctant to do anything without their say so. It can be very stressful having to be the expert in your own illness. It means you get to know all the worse things that can happen to you. It means that when in hospital you can't relax in case they stop your warfarin or don't give you enough heparin. When at home you imagine the worst when things go wrong and there's no one to turn to at times. It's very, very hard to cope with sometimes. I have had times when I've longed to have a run of the mill illness just so I could relax and stop working so hard on staying well. When on top of all of this other people look at you and say "well you're looking well," when sometimes you are feeling very ill, it can get very frustrating. Explaining what it is like to be us and just live from one day to the next never knowing how ill you will feel or whether you will be able to do something you could do yesterday is very hard to make anyone else understand.

Melissa, a member of the APLSUK e group on the internet and the Delphi forum, wrote this poem whilst feeling frustrated at the lack of understanding and difficulty getting through to others. It touched a nerve in so many of us on the internet I decided to include it in this book.

Melissa's Poem
When you come face to face with me
My symptoms may be hard to see
And you may judge and probably think...
What is this girl's disability?

My speech at times is muddled
And often it is slurred
And sometimes when I'm speaking
I can't recall a certain word

I have a tremor in my hands
That causes them to shake
I have recurrent seizures
And a devastating headache

My skin has purple blotches
My vision will often double
One day my leg will work
The next it gives me trouble

My memory is very fraught
It's really quite a shame
What a great embarrassment
To forget a face or name

Vertigo, that dreadful thing
It plagues me everyday
I can't walk straight, or heel to toe
Off balance, I tip and sway

Pins and needles crawl into my hands
But they're worse, by far, in my feet
And I've been known to just collapse
If I'm out too long in the heat

My head sometimes feels cloudy
And it's hard to concentrate
I'm so fatigued, my muscles ache
I feel I'm twice my weight

I have my blood drawn weekly
Twice when I am able
(To test a thing called INR)
Cause mine is so unstable

"You don't look sick", your comments burn
And maybe you will never learn
But if you question my disability
Spend one week of my life with me.

Written by Melissa Hoffman

There is also a wonderful website on the internet by one girl called Christine, it tells of her way of describing how she feels about Lupus to her best friend. It is called the "spoons" theory and struck a chord with many of us. Her "take" on long term illness gives others an insight into how being ill every day makes you feel. The address for this site is included at the back of this book. I would have loved to include her "theory" in this book but she may publish it herself one day so couldn't let me use it. She likens her energy to a handful of spoons (she was in a restaurant at the time!) She describes a normal day to her best friend and keeps taking a spoon away for each task she manages to do. The idea impresses on the reader how our energy only comes in a certain amount each day and once it is gone, even if it is by lunchtime we often have no reserve to draw on and have to give up. It tells how sometimes we have to decide whether to do one task or another because we know that there aren't enough "spoons" left to do both. How we never know for sure how many "spoons" we will be given each day. The whole story is far longer and more involved so I suggest everyone goes to her site and reads it. It will be sure to make you smile and nod in agreement as I did.

Chapter 6 - MS versus APS

Oh dear this argument has got me into trouble. I read a piece of research, on the internet, that suggested that up to 29% of those diagnosed with MS actually had APS. Whoops, that little piece of over enthusiastic information was going to get me a serious telling off!

Enthusiastically I joined a Multiple Sclerosis message board, eager to spread the gospel that so many of them could be saved if they just had one little blood test!

I naively thought how pleased people would be to discover they had been misdiagnosed and could be helped .I had visions of people in wheelchairs walking, as I knew had actually happened to others. I was wrong and I really learnt a lot from the angry replies I received. It stung at the time to be told I was spreading false hopes and even was asked "was I selling something?" I will confess I was very upset and confused by the reactions I received at first.

One or two people did take pity on me however and e mailed me privately to discuss the subject. We discussed the similarities and differences between the two illnesses. I found there was a lot more to Multiple Sclerosis than I had ever realised and that "magic cures" are an endless source of painful disappointment to desperate sufferers. My message made me sound like yet another "magic" cure. No wonder I triggered such an angry reaction.

The line between the two illnesses is blurred at times as Hughes Syndrome can, on occasions cause a type of demyelination (this is the gradual loss of the myelin sheath which protects the nerves). Demyelination is also the main reason for multiple sclerosis, yet in some people it can happen as part of Hughes Syndrome. The good thing about demyelination caused by sticky blood is that its progression can be stopped by anticoagulation. If you have MS there is really nothing that can actually stop this progression.

The MRI scans of the brains of two people suffering from MS and APS cannot be told apart. Is it any wonder that doctors get confused?

I find this whole subject fascinating and I really think there needs to be lots more research into both illnesses together to try to find answers to why some people appear to be suffering from both illnesses at once.

I asked Dr Hughes three questions recently. One question was "How many people diagnosed originally with MS actually have APS?" his answer was that he didn't know but possibly as many as 3% (that makes the 29% at the start of this chapter sound rather over enthusiastic).

The next question was "Do you think that if someone is found to have Hughes Syndrome they could still have MS as well? Is it likely that both illnesses would strike together?" His reply was to say it was a million to one chance that would rarely happen. It was unlikely but not impossible.

The last question was "Is there any way to tell the MRI scan of an MS patient from the MRI scan of an APS patient?" He drew me some funny little drawings of MRI scans to help me understand (I have kept them, they make me smile because he will never be an artist). He first drew two brains with white spots on them, as they would appear on the scan, both the APS brain and the MS brain had white spots randomly appearing here and there.

He then drew me another pair of brains representing MRI scans done a few months later, on these the person with MS has the spots in different places to the first scan, it is as if they are clouds moving across the sky. They may have changed size or shape as well as position. On the scan of the person with APS the white spots on the MRI scan are in exactly the same place as on the first scan, unless the person has had further mini strokes or strokes the scan will not have changed.

I have also drawn up, a list of symptoms that are the same for both MS and APS, and a list of symptoms that apply ONLY to APS and never to MS. This should help you to decide which illness is plaguing you and help any MS patients to decide whether they are one of the 3% who are misdiagnosed. It is well worth anyone diagnosed with MS asking to be tested for APS, there is nothing to lose and potentially quite a lot to gain.

Symptoms of untreated APS which are the same as MS

Sight- Blurred vision, double vision, visual disturbances (flashing lights or more complicated flickering shapes), optic neuritis, lack of eye co ordination.

Mobility- Drop foot, paralysis, clumsiness or stumbling/falling over, lack of co ordination.

Fatigue- this is extreme exhaustion with no real cause. Out of proportion to any activity undertaken.

Muscles- pain/cramps, jerking/twitching muscles, muscle spasms. Also actual chorea which is when you lose control of your movements, your body part moves without you controlling it. This could be limbs, neck, eyes, mouth, anything really.

Pain- this is often muscular aches, sometimes stiffness and joint pain, neuralgia. Sometimes sudden stabbing pains from seemingly nowhere.

Speech- may be hard to find the right words, slurred speech.

Odd symptoms such as dizziness/vertigo, pins and needles, hot or cold feelings, numbness, a burning, itching or feeling like an electric shock. You may have problems swallowing.

Memory loss and/or problems concentrating are often a problem. Your mind may suddenly freeze.

Epileptic fits, either absences or full tonic clonic fits.

Symptoms of APS which are not the same as MS

Migraine headaches often dating back to teenage years

Livedo Reticularis a pattern of blood vessels under the skin which resembles tartan

Splinter hemorrages on the nails lines usually blueish or red under the fingernail.

Fuzzy headaches which may last for days or even weeks.

Pre Eclampsia, HELLP syndrome, multiple miscarriages, stillbirths.

Blood clots causing strokes, heart attacks, pulmonary embolism, DVTs.

TIA or mini strokes

Thrombocytopenia/ low blood platelets

Anything which suggests poor circulation such as cold hands or feet.

Other signs it is APS rather than MS

Symptoms are usually improved or disappear once the blood is anticoagulated to an INR of 3 or above.

Does not respond to MS drugs such as beta interferon.

Heat does not usually make symptoms worse in most people.(though some have said it does!)

Though in untreated APS symptoms come and go there is not normally a long period with no symptoms. In other words it does not usually disappear and then return as MS does.

Incontinence is not a usual feature. Though it is possible it is not as likely as in someone with MS.

Both illnesses seem to attack mainly when a person is under 40 years of age. Both illnesses affect more women than men. Both illnesses are auto immune.
MS attacks the myelin sheath around nerves; APS attacks the blood platelets causing sticky easily clotted blood, which can strangely cause the same symptoms as MS.
In some cases APS can also affect the myelin sheath, just to confuse matters further.
The atypical MS that APS causes occurs mainly due to the brain's blood vessels becoming clogged up or perhaps even

reduced blood supply to the nerves, it seems reasonable to think that is possible. If the myelin sheath has a reduced blood supply it is not hard to imagine it could cause it to deteriorate. Thinning the blood can sometimes make dramatic improvements in the level of symptoms. It almost always reduces the symptoms in some way.

True MS as most know, is progressive with no real treatment or cure that reverses the symptoms. MS treatments usually aim at relieving symptoms or slowing down the progress of the illness. At best some treatments slow the illness down but most just help people to cope with the symptoms. Treated APS is not usually progressive so long as the anticoagulation is well managed.

MS does not usually shorten life span but APS left untreated can kill at any age.

Treatment is important for both illnesses whatever the doctors decide. Someone who has MS symptoms and a positive MRI test, plus a positive test for anticardiolipin antibodies should really consider anticoagulation. I am not suggesting that the MS diagnosis be dropped in these cases, even though that is probably what should be done. Unless it becomes obvious that this is sensible, many doctors will insist on a dual diagnosis and this is not all that important from the patient's point of view. Diagnoses are only names for symptoms so don't get worried about some doctors insisting on calling your illness APS/possible MS. Treating the APS is important from the blood-clotting viewpoint but if they insist on saying you have MS as well its not the end of the world.

In other words if you get stuck with a diagnosis of Hughes Syndrome and Multiple Sclerosis together, try not to get worked up about it. If the Hughes Syndrome is treated you will be safe from blood clots and the MS symptoms may also abate.

If you are unlucky and your MS symptoms continue then at least you are protected from the more serious and life threatening aspects of APS.

It is going to take time for research to find out exactly what is going on with these two illnesses and in the meantime all we can do is our very best to stay as well as possible and keep up to date with developments as research finds out more.

Chapter 7- 2003 was not a good year for me!

Womens stuff, not for men if they are squeamish!
It had all been very wrong for some time. For some years I'd had "womens" problems. I'd suffered long drawn out periods where I lost huge amounts of blood and was often anaemic. I'd tried the Mirena IUD which worked for a while (it is often used as it reduces the uterus lining by releasing small amounts of hormone direct to the lining). I checked that the Mirena was safe for APS patients before I agreed to try it, I would recommend that all ladies with this problem check out treatments with an APS specialist before you try them.
However, soon I was back to uncontrollable bleeding and was often reduced to just staying in the bathroom for an hour or more waiting for it to stop. The whole business became a nightmare. I spent more of the month bleeding than not. I felt weak and exhausted but still I struggled on. At work I'd be nipping to the loo every 30 minutes and going out anywhere was a logistical disaster. I soon knew where every toilet was in town and went out some days barely able to walk for the amount of padding I needed to feel secure! Of course through all this I still had APS, Sjogrens, and my angina to cope with and all of those seemed to get worse when I was bleeding. This couldn't continue and my GP said he knew I needed a hysterectomy but until my gynaecologist agreed I would have to wait. My gynaecologist was understandably nervous at the thought of operating on me. I had after all had a heart attack and had a blood clotting illness that could cause another one when he was operating. I would have been worried if he wasn't nervous!

It all came to a head in February 2003, I had 5 weeks of non stop bleeding. I saw my GP and he gave me some tablets to try. Nothing changed. The bleeding escalated until I needed to visit the toilet every 15 minutes! Whilst I won't go into too much detail for the sake of the men who may be reading this, it was terrifying. Every loo visit entailed the loss of a blood clot the size of a golf ball followed by a gush of blood. OK gentlemen, I promise that's as much detail as I'm going to go into, the gory part is now over! I think men do need to know the full horror of what can happen to us women though, as if childbirth isn't enough! Every day this went on I felt more and more ill. I went back to my GP and saw another doctor. She gave me more tablets to try, I didn't hold out much hope.

The very next day the problem was so bad that I hardly dared to walk. Just moving slightly was enough to set it off. I went back again to the GP and this time was sent to hospital. I was so relieved but even the journey there was dreadful. I sat as still as I could in my husband's car all the way, but by the time I got there I was walking like John Wayne! Every loo visit was a relief by now, as when I didn't move the blood built up inside my tummy until I was so uncomfortable that it was almost painful.

The young female doctor who examined me agreed I was in a muddle. She said she was going to have to discuss how to stop the bleeding with the other doctors but I could expect to be in hospital for some time as so many of the tablets they used in these situations were hormones which I couldn't have. She understood APS quite well I thought. She explained that warfarin was NOT the cause of the bleeding and it would have happened anyway even if I wasn't taking warfarin. I really didn't care. I remember the relief at seeing the jumbo-sized pads they had on the ward. Finally I could sleep. I hadn't slept in days as I'd been up and down all night.

The bleeding went on and on relentlessly for days while they tried out different treatments. I was getting very weak and when I went for a shower or bath in the morning I would be barely able to dry myself, I was so breathless. By about day 5 or so I was so breathless that just the short walk to the toilet and back was enough to render me speechless. One night my angina struck up in sympathy and a young doctor on night duty did his best with my help to settle it down. We discovered that a tablet that had worked once in the past could be got hold of from the general ward. I felt we were a team working out the solution together and he treated me as his equal, which is a fairly unusual and wonderful quality among doctors! He was very sweet and sat with me through the worst of the pain and gave me oxygen until the whole thing settled down. The oxygen bottle made a sound like a babbling brook and the girl in the next bed who'd had a hysterectomy that day and couldn't sleep either, said it reminded her of a water feature, we agreed it was quite relaxing! That doctor was my saviour that night, I could hear the nurses panicking about my angina and saying if he couldn't control it I would have to be moved to a general ward. He was calm and said he was confident he could settle me down. I couldn't bear the thought of being on a general ward where I knew they would keep me in bed because of the angina and there would be men as I would be in the high dependency unit which has both sexes in it.

My INR was tested daily and when I suggested I test my own INR with my machine the doctors thought it a great idea, they said I knew more about controlling my INR than they did so were happy to let me test my own and decide my own dose. The nurses were confused as to why I had such a high INR when I was bleeding. I heard one of them say "well of course she's bleeding with her INR that high." They didn't understand that with my sticky blood an INR of 3.5 wouldn't make me bleed any more than anyone else.

The next day I was so exhausted I couldn't eat, I just burst into tears at the sight of my meal. I lay on the bed really feeling detached from my surroundings and losing interest in everything. I wanted to die, yet no that's wrong, I didn't care if I died is really how I felt. I was so apathetic, I felt what would be, would be and all I wanted was to sleep and be left alone and never go to the toilet again! I knew that my three room mates were getting concerned about me but I couldn't find the energy to care.

Just as I had given up my young female doctor came in. She asked if I objected to a blood transfusion. I said no and I think I cried and told her all sorts of ridiculous things that were going around in my head. She knew this was just because I was so ill and told me to relax and I would soon start to feel better.

The blood transfusion was wonderful, I felt the life being breathed back into me as soon as it started. My nice lady doctor came and asked if I minded talking to her colleague about APS. She was training to be a haematologist and was interested to know more. She was concerned that I wasn't up to talking but I brightened immediately at the thought of being able to spout on about APS! We chatted for about half an hour and though my curtains were around my bed, the whole room of 3 other beds ended up listening to me. When she had left, my room- mates, relieved to see me livening back up told me how wonderful they thought I was to try to help others with APS. They wanted to know all about my book (which was due to be published that week). Their kind interest spurred me on and I found my strength again.

The blood transfusion was four units and took an age to go through. Sadly my toilet visits were as frequent as ever however.

My gynaecologist said " its no good putting it in at the top if its still coming out at the bottom", what a delightful turn of phrase he has!

We discussed what was to be done with me, I gave him Dr Hughes telephone number so he could ask about some of the more powerful tablets available. I told him I had, had enough and I wanted a hysterectomy. I'd swear he lost the colour in his cheeks at the thought of operating on me, though he said he would if I really wanted him to, despite me being a rather "challenging" case. Then I had a brainwave and suggested I had the hysterectomy at St Thomas Hospital as I had private health insurance. He brightened immediately and said he would ask Dr Hughes.

Soon it was all settled, I would see Mr Kenney, a colleague of Dr Hughes as soon as it could be arranged. Some strong tablets, which they hadn't dared to try yet as they promoted clotting, were given to me, hooray at last the bleeding slowed down. Dr Hughes had advised them as to what could be tried and though I still felt nervous about the tablets I really had no choice.

After a couple of weeks at home still tired but feeling far better, I went to London to see Mr Kenney. I felt safe with him straightaway. He didn't think I was a "challenging" case but an "interesting" one. He wasn't in the slightest worried about operating on me as he had Dr Hughes there as back up should there be any complications. My mind was put at rest and I waited for my hysterectomy date (in a few weeks) to come around. He explained that even with quite high INRs people with APS tend not to bleed as their blood is so sticky before anticoagulation. He said a high INR just made my blood behave in a more normal way. The cause of the bleeding was at that point thought to be a small fibroid but he said he would check it out before my hysterectomy.

In the week before my operation I began to get increasingly worried about the fact I was being told to stop taking warfarin three days before the operation. I felt that would leave me at risk of clots unless I started on heparin injections when I stopped the warfarin. I suggested this to Mr Kenney, I was full of dread that he would tell me not to be so silly. He was very supportive and told me what dose of heparin to ask for and when to start the injections, he thought it was a sensible suggestion thank goodness. Here was another one of those doctors who treat you as an equal and not as a foolish girl, it is such a relief to be treated as an intelligent person.

I was at this time avidly reading about causes of bleeding from the uterus. I found a piece of research saying that a condition called Adenomyosis was a common cause of excessive uterine bleeding, it said this was a form of endometriosis that grows inside the uterus wall. I was really fascinated when I read that it was often found in women with a high level of anticardiolipin antibodies in their blood. The description of the symptoms of Adenomyosis sounded exactly like the bleeding I had in hospital.

My GP got me started on the heparin injections, which came easily to me as I really felt I must have them to be safe. I began injecting myself with 40mg of Clexane (a brand of heparin) on the day after I stopped taking warfarin.

The day of my hospital stay dawned and my husband and I travelled down to London by train. I was to start my stay the day before the operation so they could check my INR and run through the details. My room was on the top floor overlooking the Thames, I felt relaxed and happy to be there at last.

On the day of my operation I knew I had all day to wait as it was due to take place that evening. Mr Kenney had explained he was going to do a vaginal hysterectomy as it was an easier operation to recover from. There would be no external cut or stitching so I would be in far less pain and would get over the operation more quickly. He told me to give myself the Clexane injection as normal that morning as by the time of the operation it would have worn off sufficiently. I felt safe and reassured that he was going to do his best to look after me. The nurse who was in charge of my care, hadn't been told that I was to have an injection on the day of the operation. At least if she was told she hadn't been listening. She argued with me that this wasn't the usual procedure and said he hadn't told her I was to have the injection on the day of the operation. I knew that if I insisted she would telephone Mr Kenney and find out for herself, but I knew what I had been told. I quietly gave myself an injection as soon as she left the room as I had my medications with me. I was feeling too nervous and edgy to be arguing and making a fuss that morning. I missed a chance for educating her about APS I know but even I can't face explaining all about it every time I should.

By the time it came to time to prepare for the operation I was well wound up and in an awful mood. I felt terrible as I took off all my jewellery and my nail polish. I felt sick as I put on long thrombosis stockings and an awful gown with a back opening and two dodgy ties, with no knickers! It is a dehumanising experience, which I've been through before but it doesn't get any better, especially when you know that having an operation is such a dangerous thing to do when you have APS. I knew all the horror stories from people who hadn't been looked after during operations and ended up with catastrophic APS. I also knew that bleeding though unlikely was possible during the operation. It was the usual tightrope we walk every day when we have APS, never knowing whether to be afraid of blood clots or bleeding, but magnified a hundred times over.

As I sat on the bed waiting I cried and whined at my poor long- suffering husband. He took it all and never flinched. I moaned about the hard bed, the fact I was thirsty and wasn't allowed to drink, the heat in the room, anything really. When the trolley arrived I almost leapt onto it, I was so relieved to think it would soon be over and done with.

The operation went smoothly and when I awoke I was in the recovery room and for a few moments I was in terrible pain. I remember groaning and making lots of noise, though my eyes were still closed as I felt so sleepy. Someone must have given me some morphine to shut me up because I fell straight back to sleep. The next time I came around I was warm and cosy and so comfortable, my husband found the recovery room at last and sat with me giving me sips of water. The relief that I had done it and survived this far was wonderful, I drifted in and out of consciousness for a long time. They kept me there for four hours as they wanted to be sure I was going to be alright before transferring me back to the ward. By the time I got back to the ward I was wide awake and pumping on my morphine pump with every pain. Suddenly I felt very hot and sweaty. I told the nurse on the ward , she was a large but very lovely black lady. She had a smile to light up the room and a laugh that made me want to laugh as well. She tried to rearrange my blankets but every time she unrolled me from one blanket there was another one underneath! I was like one of those Russian dolls, every layer revealed yet another one! She kept laughing and saying in her lovely accent "Whatever are dey tinkin of?" then again "Whatever are dey tinkin of?" at every blanket she removed. Finally she had pulled them all off, I think there were six in total. By now my gown was off as well and we were in fits of laughter. She made me comfy, though I was still naked as the gown was just too difficult to rearrange in the middle of the night with all the drips attached to me. Off she went with a smile and a laugh and I slept like a baby. It turned out that Mr Kenney had told the nurses in recovery to keep me warm because of my angina and they had really taken him at his word!

My recovery really went like a dream. Every day Mr Kenney visited and told me I "wasn't out of the woods yet", but that I was doing really well. I asked him what he thought had caused the bleeding? He said that my uterus was definitely abnormal and possibly it could have been a condition called Adenomyosis! He was amazed to hear that was what I had come up with as well after my research on the internet. I hope I didn't sound like too much of a know it all!

I felt I was doing well, I was walking about St Thomas' hospital by day three and even went out onto Westminster bridge to see my children on the London Eye, the weather was warm and my husband watched me carefully. Caroline from the Hughes Syndrome Foundation would meet with me and we sat out in the garden chatting. I got really used to wandering around in my pyjamas and felt so well it was wonderful.

The day I was due to leave I saw Dr Hughes and by then my first book was being sold by the Hughes Syndrome Foundation. He excitedly recommended it to the APS patient he was seeing when he spotted me in the corridor, and introduced me to her. She had lost her sight dramatically and once she had started on heparin it came back just as dramatically. He was seeing her to get her changed over to warfarin and complete the miracle.

By the time I went home I felt better than I had for months and I have to say that I am so grateful to Mr Kenney for his careful handling of my operation and aftercare. I felt pampered and very safe throughout the whole experience. I also had some wonderful nurses after my operation who made my recovery so much easier. They were really kind to me and went far beyond the call of duty with their chats and help with showering! They both received copies of my book. One was a cardiac nurse and the other a gynaecology nurse but APS affected both areas equally and they were both very interested.

I continued with injections of Clexane even once I restarted warfarin at the dose I was taking before the operation. I was sent home with smaller 20mg injections and I used them until my INR was up to 2.5. It took about a further week to get to that stage.

 I now keep 20mg Clexane by me at all times. If my INR drops below 2.5 then I use the 20mg Clexane as well until it gets back into range, this is what the doctors at St Thomas' hospital would recommend, but before my operation I had tried not to think about it as I feared the injections. The injections were easy once I got used to them and I don't mind them at all. It is surprising what you can do when you know it may save your life.

Adenomyosis was never confirmed as the cause of my bleeding but I feel that was what it was. There was no other explanation and the fibroid was so small it was unlikely it had caused the problem. I think in the future there may be some research into why Adenomyosis is more common in women with raised anticardiolpin antibodies. You can bet I will be reading any research just as soon as I find any!

Diabetes whatever next?
You would think that in one year a ten day stay in hospital in February and a blood transfusion followed by another ten day stay in a London hospital for a hysterectomy in April would have been enough wouldn't you?

No such luck! June bought more problems. I'd been so tired for such a long time, since the hysterectomy I suppose. I wasn't enjoying the wonderful summer we were having as I had no energy and a constant, dry mouth and throat (I blamed my Sjogrens for this). I also had an embarrassing problem of urgency to go to the toilet and even worse had actually wet myself a little a few times. I found this very upsetting and began to wonder if I was going to become incontinent. I also found it hard to talk to anyone about it and went back to wearing sanitary towels, which I thought I had left behind now! I hardly dared to sneeze or even laugh as I knew the outcome, and I could rarely get to the toilet in time I was always desperate.

I didn't connect all of this, my GP told me it was probably caused by my operation and to do pelvic floor exercises. I suppose I didn't really tell him how bad it had become as I really started to feel I couldn't have something else wrong with me. I was tired of things going wrong with my body and felt everyone else must be as well, even my doctor. I agreed and did my best doing huge numbers of pelvic floor exercises every day, no one could tell but sometimes I must have had a look of concentration on my face! I bought artificial saliva for my dry mouth and constantly sucked sweets and drank huge quantities of orange juice. Exhaustion I was used to and thought it must be some kind of auto immune flare up, I slept in the afternoons and missed much of the lovely summer weather. This upset me as the summer was when I "did" things, while my angina was settled. Not this summer it seemed.

I had lots of times when out with my husband on Sundays that all I would seem to do was constantly need the toilet. I think I was driving him mad and it was certainly agony for me. I couldn't enjoy going out, as I was always desperate for the toilet.

It came to a real head on an outing to the seaside with my husband. I was exhausted and really felt all I wanted to do was sit down. I dragged myself around feeling like death. I was so thirsty that I felt I could drink anything. At the same time I knew if I drank I would need the toilet.

I felt desperate and the whole day was a terrible nightmare from my perspective. I was in my favourite seaside, fishing town. It was beautiful and it was a warm sunny day. I should have been well and happy, not terrified, exhausted and needing the loo, whilst looking longingly at everyone else's drinks! As soon as I drank I wanted more, I had a thirst that couldn't be quenched. I drank anything and needed the toilet all of the time.

My ideal would have been to stay sat on the loo with a never-ending supply of drink!

At one point on that day I even looked longingly at a dog bowl filled with water that two dogs were drinking from. I was so thirsty I really would have drunk from it if no one could have seen me. I told my husband how I was feeling but made light of how bad it was, I really wanted to cry as the whole thing had taken over.

As the reader will know I am not stupid. By now I had realised something had to be wrong and I had a fair idea that it would be diabetes. I went to see my GP, he laughed and said perhaps it was an infection. I doubted it somehow. He tested my urine and was shocked to tell me I was now a diabetic. I was relieved rather than shocked, as well as a bit afraid. At least diabetes is well understood by doctors and I wouldn't have to fight for treatment this time. He told me to come back in a week and eat no sugar. He would have the blood test results by then and could start me on some medication to sort out my blood sugar.

I was dreading telling everyone that now I was diabetic as well as everything else. It was awful to see the look of disbelief mixed with pity! I get so tired of everyone having to feel sorry for me and I hate being a nuisance all the time. It felt like one more thing to settle on my shoulders and have to carry around with me.

That evening I was watering the garden and the phone rang. It was the out of hours doctor to tell me my blood sugar was 34. I was quite stupid and asked him if that was a problem. He answered that he would like me to go into hospital that evening. I told him I felt OK and couldn't I wait and see my own doctor the next day. He reluctantly agreed so long as I promised to ring him back if I felt at all unwell.

Well, the call unsettled me, I kept wondering how ill I had to feel before I got worried. My sister in law telephoned me (her daughter has been diabetic since childhood) she told me 34 was very high and she would feel better if I went to the hospital. I could hear in her voice how concerned she was. My husband looked worried and I looked at him and the kids and thought, "well how will one night in hospital hurt me?" I knew it would set everyone's mind at rest if I went and I was starting to feel afraid myself by now so I called the out of hours doctor and off to hospital I went.

Its funny but by the time I arrived my blood sugar was down to 19! My blood pressure was up but no wonder! I had a terrible night in hospital with little sleep and waited to see the doctor the next day.

The next day came and the doctor arrived. He had lots of younger doctors with him and asked me to tell them a bit about Hughes Syndrome which I did willingly.

He said, "I don't think Hughes Syndrome has a link with Diabetes though does it?" I said I didn't know but perhaps it could have an auto immune cause as everything else I have wrong is auto immune. I listed them, over active thyroid, Sjogrens syndrome , Hughes syndrome. I said it seemed likely that since everything else was connected perhaps this was as well. I was amazed to hear him say "I don't think so, I think it is most likely due to the fact Mrs Thackray is a little overweight and I suspect you like the sweeties don't you?" His entourage all smiled and nodded and generally looked pleased with their selves, the poor deluded souls!

I was amazed by this statement and tried to protest that "sweeties" were not usually a large part of my diet but I had sucked lots of them lately because of my dry mouth. I hadn't eaten any sugar at all since I found out I was diabetic. I wanted to tell him I was overweight because I couldn't exercise and in reality I didn't eat any more than anyone else. I could see this protesting would be a total waste of my effort, as he was looking so pleased with himself. I resolved to ask Dr Hughes about possible auto- immunity and let this doctor get away with it. I am 41 years old and an intelligent woman. I am successful in almost all areas of my life despite my illnesses, and being slightly overweight is the only thing I can think of that has beaten me. Being spoken to in a condescending way when you feel ill is not very nice and it hurt. Only briefly however, this nonsense was his problem, not mine. He and all doctors who belittle their patients should have a taste of being on the receiving end. One day he might be the patient, after all he will be old before me, and I only hope someone makes him feel like a stupid child. I doubt he meant to upset me, but he did. I don't drink or smoke. I do everything I should do and take care of myself well. My weight is often mentioned as an excuse for my illnesses at some stage (I ought to say I weigh slightly less than 13 and a half stone not 20!) What I want to say is "If my weight is the sole reason for me being so ill then why do I have thin friends with Hughes Syndrome who are far worse than me?" "Why do I also have so many friends who are heavier than me and are very fit and well?" It is hard enough being ill every day of your life, sanctimonious, fit and healthy people who have no way of knowing how awful that is have no right to criticise or stand in judgement EVER! The only thing it makes me want to do is rebel and go out get drunk and smoke 20 cigarettes! (Not to mention eat 20 cream cakes and a bar of chocolate!) I can't help wondering sometimes, if I did that and didn't take my tablets would I die? I don't think I'll try it just in case!

Anyway enough of my outburst, once I got home I was taking tablets for the diabetes, I stuck to the diet with no problems, no weight loss either but that's the story of my life. My blood sugar still remained high so I had some extra tablets to take the following week. The trouble was that these could send my blood sugar too low and cause me to be hypoglycaemic (low blood sugar in a diabetic can be life threatening).

This was frightening at first. I tested my blood constantly. I have had a few "hypos" now and I know the warning signs and usually take heed in plenty of time. Going out and about just needs that extra bit of organisation, I never seem to forget the diabetes, whereas when I don't have angina pain I can forget that to a degree. My confidence was knocked a little at first but I soon bounced back and got on with my life.

Going out means being sure to take my glucose monitor (if its for the day rather than a quick hour at the shops), glucose tablets, angina spray and any tablets that are due. I try to have a few biscuits or a chocolate bar handy in case I have a dip in my blood sugar. If I go away for longer I need my own medication and blood testing bag, the INR testing machine is bulky and what with spare batteries and test strips plus all my tablets, it takes up some space! I need to always be organised in order to live my life and I never know from one moment to the next when one of my ailments will strike. Every day I feel ill to some degree, whether it's just a bit dizzy, tired and achy, or a hypo in the morning followed up with an afternoon of angina! Really being ill and taking care of myself is like a part time job to me. I am my own project, keeping myself going is a daily chore that spreads itself throughout my waking hours and now and then into the night.

I do rebel a little now and then or else my life would be miserable but on the whole I have to stay as well as I can for my family's sake and my own.

The whole thing has been a learning experience, not just learning how to cope with diabetes as well as everything else. The main thing that struck me about having a common illness is the amount of support available to people with well-understood conditions such as diabetes. I received a free blood glucose monitor whilst in hospital. I had it demonstrated to me, I had diabetes explained to me in great detail. A dietician was available to advise on the right foods to eat.

What a contrast to being told I had Hughes Syndrome. I was told nothing then except the name of the test that was positive. I had to discover everything else for myself. If I hadn't done that I had a 50/50 chance of having another blood clot. How many blood clots would I have had to have before I got the correct treatment I wonder?

Imagine if diabetics were treated that way. No advice, no free monitor just hope for the best! Imagine if they all had to search on the internet for a doctor and to find out what diabetes was. Imagine living with diabetes if every time you were ill you needed to explain to the doctor exactly what diabetes was and how it affected you because you knew more about it than him. What if you were left to fend for yourself with diabetes as many people are with Hughes syndrome? Oh guess what? I know what would happen. People would be made disabled in droves, they would die without anyone knowing why, legs would be amputated and people would become blind, heart attacks and strokes would be commonplace. Does this sound like anything familiar? Perhaps 100 years ago a diabetic would have been in the same situation that a Hughes syndrome patient, often finds themselves in now. The wonderful treatment I receive for my diabetes had made me more determined that Hughes Syndrome should have the same level of understanding and treatment as soon as possible.

Even now I see the nurse regularly at my GPs surgery to discuss my blood sugar control and even to just chat if I feel down. Now there's a novelty! Even once you have seen the right doctor and got the right treatment there is no one you feel you can turn to when you have Hughes Syndrome and feel sad or afraid or worried. The chances are the nurse won't understand what the illness is and by the time you've explained you are exhausted. Your GP has referred you to a specialist because he doesn't understand the intricacies of Hughes Syndrome. Your specialist is many miles away and a busy man. Who can you turn to? The answer is that the only people you can tell who can help are other people who live with Hughes Syndrome. I think the level of support for diabetics is wonderful and needed, I just wish that same level of support were available for Hughes Syndrome. Perhaps we will get there, one day? The Hughes Syndrome Foundation is working hard to raise awareness but it really is a struggle.

Dr Hughes did explore the possibility of my diabetes being auto immune but there is no evidence of it. I refuse however to believe there is no connection at all. My parents are both fit and well with no signs of diabetes type 2, there is no diabetes type 2 in my family's history that anyone has heard of, even though some were over weight. On the other hand my brother has type 1 diabetes that is auto immune. The difference between Dr Hughes and the other doctor was that Dr Hughes listened to me and thought I had made an intelligent suggestion. He investigated my suggestions and didn't make me feel foolish, just sensible.

Well as I write this it is still 2003, so there is still time for something else to go wrong I guess, but ever optimistic I will tell myself I have had more than my share and I'm coping. Some days only just coping but mainly I cope and life is still worth living. I still laugh and I still dance and sing to the radio and embarrass my children, so I know all is alright with the world.

As a last mention of my personal life, in early 2004 my husband discovered he had advanced bowel cancer which though treatable was not curable.

The stress of this affected me so badly that I felt I was in danger of not looking after my own health, so I succumbed to some tablets to reduce my anxiety which I still take. I have found that APS and terrible stressful and deeply distressing life events can co exist, though I don't recommend it! I have managed very well and surprised myself by how much my body can manage when it has to.

At the start I wondered how on earth I would cope and panicked about letting everyone down, but by taking one day at a time I am fine. I think in the coming days I will need all my strength to help my darling husband and from somewhere I seem to find it over and over again. I am so relieved that I found Dr Hughes when I did and got my illnesses treated and under control. I have no time to be ill now and think far less about what "may" happen to me than I ever have. Seeing my husbands strength of character when he knows what he knows, drives me on.

I previously felt sorry for myself so often because I have to live with multiple illnesses but now I know that while there is life there is hope and if you have APS there is a huge amount that can be done to help you. We are very lucky to be alive and if we are careful we may quite easily die of old age. However hard it seems, remember we have that all important hope and so many, like my husband have none.

Enjoy every moment that you can!

Chapter 8- Depression and Anxiety

This is going to be a terrible chapter for me to try to write. I will thank my friend Judi Page in advance as she is often struck down by depression and I will ask her to check I haven't said entirely the wrong thing. I have also included her thoughts on depression in this chapter.

I am not completely ignorant of what depression feels like. I think I have been there and managed to claw my way out without anti depressants. I do think however that my experience of depression was tempered by the fact I have a loving family around me constantly pushing me onwards and slowing my downward spiral. I also have a naturally optimistic nature when it comes to my illness. I am known for always smiling, I think some may even find me irritatingly cheerful at times! I always feel that I go into hospital to be made well, and I always feel that if I take care of myself I will be fine.

I feel as though I know that whatever life throws at me I can cope and won't be beaten by it, but even then from time to time things do beat me and that is very hard to admit.

Possible reasons for depression
Of course ill people are often depressed, it is understandable if your life is restricted and frustrating. However in the case of someone with APS this may not be the only reason for depression. Depression can occur because of physical damage to the area of the brain that controls emotions. This can mean that a previously, cheerful person can find themselves uncharacteristically sad and tearful all the time for no good reason. It can also mean that a previously good- natured type

can become more aggressive. I know some people have been amazed at their own behaviour, knowing this isn't how they usually react.

It is important to remember that restricted or poor blood flow to the brain can cause depression. It is possible for a mental state to be caused by a physical problem. If there is no permanent damage then it is possible that thinning the blood will cure the problem.

Things to try if you feel down
Talk to someone, anyone sympathetic will do, often a doctor or nurse who doesn't need you to protect them from your real feelings.

Get out of the house if possible. Going out and about can lift a black mood.

Do something you love like painting, writing or curl up in front of the TV with a box of chocolates!

Pamper yourself with a manicure, hairdo or something indulgent. If money is short have a girly night like you did as a teenager! (apologies to the men, you know the sorts of things men like to do!)

Don't bottle up your feelings, if you are cross then let it out! Your close friends and family need to know if they are irritating you to death!

Talk to others who have the same problems you have. Join a support group on the net.

Feeling anxious over a long period of time can mean you become depressed. If something is worrying you then discuss it with your doctor or someone who knows more about it than you. Knowledge can make you feel less anxious. Often the worry becomes less of a problem once its been discussed.

Try not to be alone too much. Being alone means time to think too much. I am beginning to think that thinking too deeply about the problems in your life too often can depress you.

Don't allow others to drive you to depression. I know this is possible from experience. If there is someone in your life that constantly drags you down, then stop allowing them to do it. Be determined that you will be be surrounded only by those who care about you and make you feel happy. People who upset you must be avoided as being upset will often trigger your illness to go up a notch or two. If you cut out the negative people from your life (that's relatives as well as so-called friends!) you may avoid depression and improve your general well being. Living with Hughes syndrome means getting through each day is enough of a challenge, stick to people who help you get through. Lose anyone who drags you down and tell them why if you feel up to it!

This is also the time that alternative therapies can be useful to keep your spirits up. Nothing that can be swallowed in the way of alternative medicine is advisable without checking with your doctor. However, things such as reflexology, aromatherapy, massage etc can be very helpful. I don't profess to know whether they do actually work at all but the main thing is whether they make you feel better and happier. Make sure the therapist knows your full medical history so that they know to be gentle and not cause any bruising. Some may ask you to ask your doctor if it is safe for you to have their treatment. Usually it will be fine but just have common sense i.e. don't go for accupuncture if you are taking warfarin, not that its likely you would have any serious problem with bleeding, just that it could be rather messy! The therapists are usually very good at talking and listening to people after all it is part of their job so they probably won't mind you telling them some of your troubles. At the end of the day if you leave feeling relaxed and better than when you arrived it is helping you.

OK I know that "real" depression is not that easy

I know that once real depression sets in then nothing will help. Feelings of despair and hopelessness take over and life seems hardly worth the effort any more.

If this is you, then seek help. Don't keep it in, tell your doctor, take anti depressants if he thinks it will help you. There is no shame in admitting you have a problem. For goodness sake other people get depressed when they have no other illness to deal with, you have the right to help! When depressed it is usually far easier to hide away, than seek help but seek it you must. Life is still good and you just need some help to see that, don't ever feel that depression equals failure. Anti depressants can make you more able to cope with your life and that has to be good.

My experience of depression.

In the long dark days before diagnosis I remember the hopeless feeling of waking up to another awful day full of weird symptoms and exhaustion. I remember how I struggled to keep going in my normal routines and failed time and time again. Every day was an uphill hopeless struggle and no one on god's earth understood or could help. The smallest criticism could leave me a quivering sobbing wreck. I had many days where I had begun to think that the whole thing was far, far too much for me to bear. I kept going because I had young children and they needed me but I know I was getting very snappy with them. My poor daughter would have a friend to stay and I would endlessly lose my temper over little things like an untidy bedroom. I felt so ill that it took all my effort to look after my own family, when they had friends to stay it felt like a major problem! I find it hard to remember how it felt now as my natural instinct is to have all their friends to stay and enjoy their company. The experience that

I had of depression was that it felt like I was falling into a deep dark well and I kept crawling up to the top but it kept getting harder and harder to do. My biggest fear was letting go and dropping in as I wasn't sure what would happen if I gave in.

No one else knew about the well except me. Some days I was further down and others I nearly got out but one careless comment could send me back in. Every kind and understanding word or sweet thing done for me would make me fight on. Every unkind comment or bad day of feeling ill would send me back down.

There is also the small case of a slight hallucination or delusion I used to have, I guess that is what you call it? I never have talked about it but if it helps someone else then here goes. Whenever I rested on my bed, as I needed to do each afternoon, I would hear a small aeroplane overhead. It sounded like a model plane or some very light aircraft buzzing in the sky. It always seemed to be there when I laid on my bed. In my confused mind I started to think that perhaps the aeroplane or something in it was making me ill! It sounds so crazy now but then it made sense to me. I knew others would find that a very odd thing to say though, so I never told a soul about this delusion. I can laugh at the thought of me even beginning to think such a silly thing now but at that time it was real. So much of this depression was hidden. No one knew I felt like this and I was too afraid to try to tell anyone. In fact I angrily denied depression to my consultant and my GP.

It was only once I had my heart attack that my mental health returned to normal. The pressure of being alone and no one understanding how ill I felt, was suddenly lifted from my shoulders. Everyone has heard of a heart attack and it was now obvious that I was ill and needed help. People were kind and did their best to make my life easier. The sense of relief instantly made me feel a hundred times better.

Even now though, depression has a habit of trying to sneak into my life. When I was first told I had diabetes, it tried to come back. I had my first "hypo" (low blood sugar) and I got very down about having another illness to deal with. It just got worse and worse over a week. I hated everyone and had a rage inside me against everyone who had a normal life. It came to head when I went to an opening of a computer suite at a local school, with my daughter. Everyone seemed so happy and carefree. I felt like I was the odd one out and none of these stupid people knew what it was to live in my awful body.

It was all completely unreasonable, but I think if one of those "happy people", had said one single wrong word to me I'd have exploded! As it was I kept making unpleasant remarks under my breath which caused my daughter to look at me in a quizzical manner now and then. Every petty little problem anyone told me about made me boil up inside, "how could they find minor upsets such a problem when I had all this to deal with?" I hated feeling like this, I couldn't face people easily I wanted to hide away so I didn't have to listen in case they said something that set me off. If I did anything wrong at home, I felt myself daring my husband or children to complain, I was ready to fly off the handle if they did. It came to an end when I saw the nurse at my GPs surgery for a routine diabetes check up. I told her I couldn't tell her about how I felt without crying. She got the tissues down. She listened as I poured it all out and told me it was understandable to feel this way. I had been through a lot and it was normal to feel so angry about it. She asked if I needed anti depressants to help me through but I said no. As soon as I let it all out the depression lifted! It was like magic! I now know how to make it go away. Telling someone who is sympathetic helps me. It has to be someone I don't need to protect from my true feelings, as I can't burden those I love with this without feeling guilty. Feeling guilty then makes me more depressed!

The other thing that I have found relieves my depression is writing about what is happening to me. Also just writing about anything always cheers me up and sets me on the right road.

I now try to nip sad thoughts in the bud. The moment I feel myself getting negative about my situation I try to do something that will help me. I go shopping if the weather is good and buy something new to wear or get my hair done. I sit at my computer and write for a while. If I felt it was getting serious I would go and have a good cry with my friendly nurse again, now that I know she doesn't mind. If I ever get badly depressed again I will consider anti depressants but I still haven't lost that fear of "giving in and letting it get the better of me". Even though I tell everyone reading not to be ashamed I find it hard to take my own advice. I think even my GP would be surprised to read this chapter and know how I really felt, I keep it so well hidden!

Most of the time I am happy and positive but my word, illness can drag anyone down.

Judi Page, who has APS, Syndrome X angina, Sjogrens and mild lupus amongst one or two other things to cope with, has sent me a great deal of information from her experiences of depression here are her thoughts in her own words

Depression from Judi's viewpoint
Depression is not fatal, although on occasion it may make you wish that it were so.

Depression is NOT the cause of your illness, indeed it may be a physical symptom of the brain reacting to the abnormal blood supply produced by Hughes Syndrome.

Depression is not unusual in people with Hughes Syndrome even when it is not an actual symptom of the blood disorder. The depression can arise as one of the effects of having a long-term illness especially one which has restricted your lifestyle and made even everyday tasks a big effort not leaving you with much energy to do the things you enjoy. Also you may have had Hughes for a long time and had difficulties getting diagnosed. This will have caused a lot of stress for you, which in the long term may have turned into depression.

You need treatment for Hughes Syndrome but don't turn away from ALSO taking anti-depressants if depression is one of your problems. I used to be very much against taking these pills, I thought I ought to be able to 'cure' my depression without resorting to tablets. One of my doctors taught me to look at them in a different way. If you cut your leg badly you put a plaster on to help while your body heals the wound. In the same way you can use anti-depressants as a 'plaster' for the mind to help with the recovery from the depression.

Normally I have a very good sense of humour, so good that it has been known to get me into trouble for not appearing to take things seriously. I am known for always having a ready smile. But there are times when I suffer from depression although I can be very good at hiding these feelings from others. I used to feel that there was something shameful in having depression, other people got through life without it and many people had much harder lives than I did so I felt that I had no right to be depressed. I know better now. A lot of people suffer from depression and it isn't something to feel a failure about. It is also something that is poorly understood by people who haven't had it, they think you can just 'pull yourself together' or 'snap out of it' or they think you just need to have a holiday or need to get out more. They really don't understand that this depression doesn't work like that. It's like trying to explain a migraine to someone who has only ever had headaches. They can only relate to the times when they have felt sad, miserable, fed-up, over-tired or have been grieving for a loss of a person or a particular lifestyle. Having Hughes Syndrome will mean that you feel all of these things but depression goes further and deeper.

My personal episodes of depression have been in two very different forms. The first was an acute form, which I suffered after having had pneumonia badly. I really did feel like I was going to fall into a big black bottomless pit mentally, there was this big weight pushing me down. I felt as though I was on the very edge and if I fell in I would never get out again. It was terrifying and I just couldn't stop crying. I didn't understand what was happening to me. I lived alone and had no one in the house to talk to or to reassure me. I was so frightened I phoned my GP as I couldn't think what else to do. She kindly saw me straight away and talked to me for about half an hour until I felt I could cope again. I started taking anti-depressants and saw a counsellor for twenty minutes a week for a couple of months just to make sure I was still doing OK and to give me some support.

But the type of depression that I normally get with Hughes Syndrome has happened on a few occasions. It is more a feeling of being constantly dragged down, it is much milder than the feelings I had with the other type of depression but goes on day after day and I can just sink lower and lower. Sometimes I would cry for no reason, I would be doing something and tears would just start falling. Everything becomes difficult to deal with, even small problems are hard to solve and decisions are hard to make. Everyday life seems to be a constant battle and nothing goes easily. Sometimes it is difficult to see the purpose of my life. I have no husband or children and live alone, I have a lot of pain, I cannot go out much and I don't have any money. On bad days I have sat there and wondered why I carry on.

Again I have taken anti-depressants. They have not made me happier but have made me feel mentally stronger and much more able to cope with everyday problems and decisions. I try to find small things which I enjoy even it is only a bar of chocolate or looking at a beautiful sunset for a couple of minutes. This doesn't cure the depression but it can give a temporary relief so at least you have a break from the constant dragging. My friends also help not just by providing support but by being there to talk to. When I talk to my friends I try not to be depressed, I try to stay light hearted and cheerful even when I'm feeling down. I find the more I can pretend to be cheerful then the more likely I am to actually be cheerful. I know that my friends have problems of their own too and they don't always want to have my depression off-loaded onto them although I know that they will be there if I really need them. I like to share their problems also, they are my friends and I want to help them but also knowing that I am not the only person with problems helps me not to feel isolated and unconnected. Feelings of isolation and of not being connected to the rest of the world are often associated with depression and I think it's important to try to fight back. Some of my friends have admitted that they find it difficult to know what to say to me when I am depressed. That's very easy to answer. Talk to me about anything. I don't need you to talk to me about my depression very often, I will tell you if I do, but talk to me about your life, keep me involved with what is going on, make me feel a part of things.

So am I depressed?

To help you work out whether you are depressed go through the following list and see how many of them apply to you.

Poor concentration, loss of pleasure in life, feeling alone, loss of interest including loss of interest in sex, feeling guilty or worthless, loss of confidence, feeling inadequate, having low self esteem, losing interest in your appearance, thinking about death or suicide. It's scary how many of those apply when you have an illness to cope with isn't it?

Other signs are a withdrawal from life, not feeling you can be bothered to do things and avoiding people. Some become angry and quick tempered at others or at themselves. Crying a lot is common when depressed, often for no apparent reason or for a trivial reason. You may feel you can't do things you were previously good at and make mistakes.

The types of things we may do to cope with all of this vary. Some drink to excess or smoke more. Getting agitated and crying a lot may somehow relieve the pressure for others. Some find anger and shouting a release, others withdraw and hide away from life. In extreme depression people even harm themselves either causing injuries or even suicide.

The important thing is to recognise what is happening to you before you get to the stage of feeling life has nothing to offer. Seeking help is the only real way out of depression. Never ever be ashamed of being depressed, just be sure to look for help sooner rather than later. Remember when people feel ill they all get down or depressed by it. It's just normal!

Chapter 9
Wendy - The reason why we should all fight for the right treatment

It was either late 2002 or early 2003 when Caroline at the Hughes Syndrome foundation told me that someone who needed help and advice had contacted her. The contact was from the very worried husband of a lady who had Hughes Syndrome. She felt that I might be better placed to talk to him as I actually had Hughes Syndrome and she knew that he lived in the area of my support group.

She gave me his telephone number and warned me that it sounded as though he and his wife had been through awful, awful times.

I have to say it was with some trepidation that I telephoned him, I didn't know what to expect, how ill his wife was or whether I could help. I felt I might be rather inadequate but was determined to try to be of use if I could.

I listened as Jim told me all about his poor wife Wendy. The terrible things she had been through and was still going through. I felt I might cry but refused myself that luxury as Jim was being so strong.

Wendy had, had this mystery illness for many years, really since at least the 80's when APS was first being discovered. She had not had a proper diagnosis initially and then when she did develop blood clots and got a diagnosis of Hughes syndrome she was given warfarin, only to have it later withdrawn. Jim and Wendy had no reason to question her treatment, this was in the 80's and 90's and APS was even less understood or even known of, than it is now. She went through many operations, some of which could have been avoided. The operations combined with the withdrawal of warfarin caused Wendy to develop what he now knew to be catastrophic APS. She had many, many clots, she had three strokes and nine blood clots just in her chest and neck.

Wendy was left in a terrible state, even at this late stage her INR was not being adequately controlled. She ended up confined to bed, unable to move, she had one arm amputated as it was full of clots cutting off her circulation. She was in constant pain and the whole situation had turned into one huge nightmare for both Jim and Wendy. He was careful to tell me that she tried to be cheerful and had a wonderful sense of humour but was unable to do anything for herself.

I was at a loss to know what to tell Jim to do. I suggested he got an INR machine and regulated her INR himself as he felt it was still not adequately monitored. He said he would try but as Wendy's circulation was so poor and she only had one hand to try for blood it might be difficult. I asked if she could get to Dr Hughes at St Thomas hospital. I knew the answer really, she was too ill to travel.

Dr Hughes was instead going to be able to advise doctors at a local hospital where she would soon be going to be evaluated. I told Jim that there was some hope and he shouldn't give up, but his honest reply stunned me. He told me that he very much doubted that anything could be done for Wendy now and if I had seen her I would understand why he said that. I told Jim how sorry I was and we had a long chat about how terrible it all was and what a terrible shame that Wendy hadn't had the help she needed at an earlier stage of her life.

I had heard quite a few "miracle" stories of people in wheelchairs walking and people having their vision restored when their Hughes Syndrome was treated. However I had never heard what happened to people as seriously ill and damaged by APS as poor Wendy was. I really felt out of my depth and thought that perhaps Jim was right about her prognosis.

I came off the phone about an hour later feeling that I really hadn't helped at all. I also felt upset as hearing all of this when you have the illness yourself is distressing but I knew I was being treated correctly so didn't feel afraid. Later that evening Jim and Wendy's daughter contacted me by e mail. It was a lovely note thanking me for helping her dad and saying how talking to me had meant a lot to him. I was so pleased to think that just listening and understanding had made a difference, however small.

Jim and I talked on one other occasion and I felt I'd upset him by talking about his problems, as he had a few tears and couldn't speak for a little while. I do think though that perhaps talking to me was helping him in some small way even though he had got a little upset. His daughter still kept in touch and we sent each other e mails. Then one day I got the e mail I had dreaded. Wendy had died. Though she had suffered and in that situation death is a relief as well as a loss, I still felt sad to think of Jim all alone. She was just 56 years old.

After a little while I telephoned Jim again. He wanted to know if I knew anyone who needed an INR machine. I did and though it hadn't been much help to Wendy I know the person who ended up with it has made good use of it.

He told me that he had collected Wendy's ashes and managed to make us both laugh with a few quite macabre jokes, which he told me Wendy would have found hilarious. He told me he had insisted that the cause of death be recorded as Antiphospholipid Syndrome despite some opposition from the doctors concerned. I felt very proud of him for insisting on that at such a time. Even though Jim was obviously going through a very hard time he only faltered once when talking to me of Wendy's suffering and quickly regained his composure. This dignified man had borne far more than most of us are called upon to bear and I felt sure that Wendy was watching and feeling very proud. I know I couldn't help much but I tried my best and I knew Jim and his daughter appreciated that. I vowed that for Wendy's sake that whenever I heard someone say on the internet forums that their doctor was going to take them off warfarin I would speak up and tell them what happened to Wendy. I have used her story often to convince people how important it is to push for treatment and never stop pushing.

I thought that perhaps this was a rare case, a "one off". I knew of one other person who had her leg amputated but she was the only other amputee I had come across.

I was mistaken. Later in 2003 I was contacted first by a man whose sister in law had both legs amputated and later by the lady herself. In her case again it was caused by withdrawal of warfarin. It seems that giving an APS patient warfarin and then later withdrawing it is more likely to set off catastrophic APS than never having the warfarin at all! I have supported this second lady and tried to advise her the best I can. She knows where I am if she ever needs me and I really hope that now she will be sure that she is treated correctly. How terrible to be given the correct treatment, be on safe ground, and then because one doctor thinks that warfarin is unnecessary and withdraws it, you lose both legs! How can this be right? There really needs to be guidelines in place for all doctors who are treating people who have Hughes Syndrome. The present situation, 20 years after this was all discovered, is appalling and needs to change.

These two ladies both live not too far from me. I have another support group member who had warfarin withdrawn but had less dramatic but still unnecessary problems. If I have found three such people in my corner of the world without even looking, how many more are out there? How many more people are unaware of the danger they are in? It is bad enough that people with Hughes Syndrome are constantly denied the treatment they need or even the blood tests needed to diagnose them, to give them the correct treatment and then take it away is beyond belief! The only way this will change is if the doctors are educated about Hughes Syndrome and its treatment. It seems that this takes time and I am impatient to get the message to all doctors.

Until this happens I urge everyone reading this book to take the time to check your INR regularly and record it. Have your latest INR results always at hand. Take this illness seriously and be sure to take your tablets. Never allow anyone to withdraw your warfarin. If you need surgery be sure that you have a sensible regime such as I describe when talking of my hysterectomy, in place before you ever get to the operating theatre. If you feel your doctor doesn't understand APS then either try to educate them if they are open to that or go elsewhere. Never let anyone do anything to you that you feel is not right. Get a Medic alert bracelet and have your APS doctor listed. Have a list of your conditions and medication ready should you need to go into hospital along with a telephone number for your APS specialist and a note of your target INR and how important it is to keep it in range. There are four main causes of catastrophic APS, these are, oral contraceptives, withdrawal of warfarin treatment, operations (including "minor" procedures, anything invasive can cause problems), and infections (not just any old infection but the more serious stuff). Infections must be avoided, where possible, and if they happen, treated aggressively with antibiotics before they get out of control. We need to know those causes well and we need doctors to know them as well.

Wendy and others like her must not have died in vain, my other lady must not have lost her legs for nothing. At least if their experiences make you take care and be stronger about your treatment there will have been some good coming from their terrible misfortune.

Remember that if you do everything you can to look after yourself there is far more chance that you will stay well than develop anything awful. This is not about frightening you but making sure you know how serious APS is and how important it is to take care of yourself at all times. The horror stories almost always come because people haven't had the correct treatment for their sticky blood. With the correct treatment and careful monitoring the vast majority of people with APS do very well.

 I wish that it wasn't necessary to tell horror stories in order to make people take notice but it is at this moment in time. Once we can sit back and feel that doctors can be trusted to know how to look after us we won't need to have Wendy in the back of our mind. Until that happens it is perhaps for the best that her story drives us on to be sure that everything is done correctly for us at all times.

Chapter 10 - So What's new?

As Hughes Syndrome is a relatively "new" disease more and more is discovered about the processes involved in sticky blood and how it can be controlled all the time.

The only way to make new discoveries is for the clever people to conduct trials and do research. There is always a huge amount of research underway at St Thomas hospital,London, if the funds were limitless there would be a whole lot more as there is so much yet to be explained about this illness.
Dr Hughes and his team work in both the clinic and the laboratory. The combination of seeing real patients and discussing their real problems and working in the laboratory is a rare situation. It is a great strength for the team to be able to discuss the findings in the laboratory and compare them with what they discover from their patients.
All of the following is being researched at the Rayne Institute, St Thomas hospital.

Many areas of the body can be affected by Hughes syndrome and many previously mysterious health problems can be explained by the poor blood supply caused by sticky blood.
The brain is the main area affected by sticky blood. There is research into the reasons why the brain is affected more often and more dramatically in many patients.
The kidneys need a blood supply as much as any other part of the body. If the supply is reduced by clotting (or perhaps narrowing in the arteries), then high blood pressure can result. It may be that thinning the blood with warfarin could

reverse the high blood pressure problem or at least improve it. Of course untreated APS can mean that some people have more permanent damage to their kidneys but if people are treated early enough perhaps high blood pressure could be resolved? The results of research into APS and high blood pressure caused by sticky blood affecting the kidneys has so far shown that most show an improvement if their INR is kept above 3.

Immunoglobins are a relatively experimental treatment at the moment. They work by suppressing the immune system. This is a treatment given intravenously and is very expensive. However it has been shown to be useful for some of the people resistant to the usual treatments. Warfarin works for most patients but some people still clot and it is useful to have something else to try.

Headaches are the most common symptom of APS. Whether it's migraine, "a fuzzy head" or sharp stabbing pains, just about everyone who has Hughes syndrome will know all about headaches! It has been known for many years that some migraine sufferers are more at risk of having a stroke. It would surely make sense to test migraine sufferers for Hughes syndrome as a matter of course? There is active study ongoing into the connections between migraine and sticky blood.

Negative blood tests are another worry for people who totally fit the clinical description of Hughes Syndrome and respond very well to anticoagulation but just cannot seem to have a positive blood test! The answer to this is most likely to be that the present tests are imperfect and there are perhaps other antiphospholipid antibodies involved. Some of these people test positive for Anti beta 2 glycoprotein-I and yet negative for the usual blood tests. At St Thomas hospital a person with classic symptoms such as multiple blood clots or miscarriages but negative blood tests would usually have the chance of trying anticoagulation. Such patients are carefully studied by the team. It is to be hoped that they can find answers as it must be the most distressing situation to be in such danger but have no proof. I remember my relief at my positive blood test and if the tests can be refined so that all APS patients can feel that relief it will be wonderful. It would seem there could be many sub sets of APS patients, those who test negative but have all the symptoms, those who only clot in pregnancy, those who have arterial clots, those with venous clots, some who test positive, have MS symptoms, but never actually have a clotting incident. There are many many more I could think of. In time tests will be found that identify everyone with APS but it will take time.

For those of us treated with warfarin there is no doubt that self testing our INR can be a huge step to taking control of our bodies and preventing the symptoms we suffer from. Those with an INR that jumps up and down, seemingly for no reason, benefit from regular testing and adjustments to the dose of warfarin. A close management of warfarin and INRs can only be achieved through self testing more often than clinics are able to do.

Poor INR control leads to more blood clots which is both terrible for the patient and expensive to treat. Good control of the INR can mean a relatively "normal" life for many people with APS. As an example I find my angina is fine when my INR is over 4 but not so good below 4. Without experimenting a little and self testing my INR I would never have found this out.

At St Thomas hospital they are trying to show that self testing should be the norm for Hughes Syndrome patients taking warfarin by exploring the cost effectiveness of this approach. Self testing is relatively inexpensive compared to treating multiple blood clots.

In some of the patients with Hughes syndrome there seems to be a tendency for artery disease at a relatively young age. It has become clear that some of the antibodies measured when testing for Hughes syndrome may have a direct effect on the arteries. This is something that causes great interest in medical circles as it is yet another contributing factor to "clogged" arteries (or in their terms atheroma!)

Seizures are a well known symptom of Hughes Syndrome. However it is not something that is routinely tested for in epilepsy clinics. APS is a major cause of "fits" and more research is needed to find out how many epileptics could be suffering from Hughes syndrome and could be treated with anticoagulants.

Statins are a group of well-known drugs used for reducing cholesterol. Work completed by the team at St Thomas Hospital, with another team in Milan, showed that statins also have a "calming" effect on the lining of blood vessels.
This is of huge significance for Hughes Syndrome. As the illness affects both the vessels and the blood flowing through them "calm" blood vessels can only be helpful!

There is some kind of genetic link involved in Hughes Syndrome. Often it is more a case of "clusters" of family members having the illness than a definite pattern. There are collaborations between the team at St Thomas' and several other worldwide groups to try to find out more about the genetics involved in Hughes Syndrome.

Since both Hughes syndrome patients and Lupus patients are seen at the clinic at the hospital the team are well placed to study the links between the two illnesses. 1 in 5 Lupus patients develop Hughes syndrome, however it seems a rarity for a Hughes syndrome patient to develop Lupus. By comparing patients and hearing first hand the problems caused by having both illnesses the doctors are in a great position for working out how the links between the illnesses work.

Sjogrens syndrome is yet another autoimmune illness that seems to go along with APS. Dry eyes and mouth along with mild lupus is the description of Sjogrens and many people with APS seems to have this problem. This is another one of the links that is studied.

St Thomas hospital are in a great position to look at the cost effectiveness of various treatments for Hughes syndrome. This can be a benefit to patients needing proof that they need a certain treatment as sadly with both the NHS and insurance companies cost versus effectiveness are often considered before the actual patients needs.

When it comes to the group in the "grey" area who may need warfarin but no one is sure as they haven't had a so called "clotting incident", there is a problem deciding between either aspirin or warfarin as a treatment.
St Thomas' is co ordinating an international study into the effectiveness of warfarin versus aspirin over 5 years. Hopefully this will lead to a better understanding of which treatment people should "go" for.

It is not just research in the laboratory of course. It is becoming apparent that sticky blood can cause reduced blood flow to heart muscle in some causing angina.

In others it is obvious that there is a problem with the blood flow to the digestive system causing any number of different digestive symptoms, from cramps to indigestion. The breadth of illness that can be caused by having sticky blood is seemingly endless. Blood travels to and is needed by, every organ of the body; even the skin is affected by livedo and ulcers to name only a couple of possibilities. Only by seeing large numbers of patients with Hughes syndrome can doctors find out the seemingly limitless symptoms that can be attributed to this illness.

Be reassured that this is just a selection of studies and research into this perplexing illness. There is so much happening all over the world in laboratories and clinics. In the future there will be new treatments and far more people diagnosed with Hughes syndrome. By the time we are old I am sure that Hughes syndrome will be viewed as a common and well understood illness, all thanks to the people who find our illness fascinating enough to try to work out why and how and all the other questions we need answers for.

Chapter 11- Internet sites

http://www.hughes-syndrome.org/
This is the home page of the Hughes Syndrome Foundation (HSF). It is "the" place for up to date information, newsletters etc. I recommend that everyone should join wherever they live.
Hughes Syndrome Foundation
Louise Coote Lupus Unit,
Gassiot House,
St Thomas Hospital,
London.
SE1 7EH

Telephone 020 7188 8217

E mail hsf@btconnect.org

http://apls.tk/
This is the home of Eddies survey and information pages. His extensive survey reveals a lot of less well known symptoms and what percentage of people have them. It makes interesting reading and you may find out that something you hadn't connected with Hughes Syndrome is actually just another symptom! I would urge everyone to have a go at filling in the survey as the more replies he gets , the more accurate the picture of APS it shows. Eddie has APS and is a mine of information for all those who visit the APLSUK site.

http://www.butyoudontlooksick.com/spoons.htm
This is the spoons theory I previously mentioned in this book. It refers to Lupus but would apply to any long term illness really. I thought it was a great way of explaining things.

http://www.myida.org/lookgood.htm
A website to read if people are always telling you how "well" you look when you feel awful! You are NOT alone!

http://health.groups.yahoo.com/group/aplsuk/
Lynette's site which I also moderate on with an international team. This is the best support group in my humble opinion and attracts the most members (over 700 I think). It is well moderated with a light hand and no decisions ever taken lightly. It is a place to discuss problems, chat, tell jokes, and ask questions. You will always get an answer or 10 here.

http://forums.delphiforums.com/APShelp/start
This is a forum I have set up myself in an attempt to recreate the old Delphi forum. A friend of mine Mark Waxman, set up the original Delphi forum to help others. Sadly he was unable to run it, handed it over to someone else and the forum was closed down soon after. As this is the place where a lovely lady called Sandy once told me to "get it sorted out, this disease can cause terrible problems and you don't need any of it", I was heart broken to find it had been closed down. The Delphi forum was where I found out all about Hughes Syndrome and ended up helping others. My writing really began because I could see so many of the same questions being asked on this forum and felt a book from our (the patients) point of view was needed.
Though with my husband ill I thought I couldn't manage to run a forum I am enjoying the distraction. Opting out of the world of APS support is not really an option for me now or in

the future. If I am temporarily unable to support others there is no doubt in my mind that as soon as I am able I will be right back there. I enjoy it too much to drop out for any length of time. I try to visit as often as I can to check if anyone needs any help. Anyone can contact me through this forum. If I am able I will answer.

A final note- This book is written from my own and others experiences of Antiphospholipid or Hughes Syndrome. It is intended to work as if it were a good and knowledgeable friend you can turn to for sensible and easy to understand answers to the many questions you have. It is not a medical book and I am not medically trained. In no way should this book be used in place of your doctor at any time. It is full of my personal opinions and information, which I believe to be true from my own research and speaking to other APS patients. That knowledge is no substitute for proper medical help and I would never suggest it was.

Printed in the United Kingdom
by Lightning Source UK Ltd.
107076UKS00001B/154-204